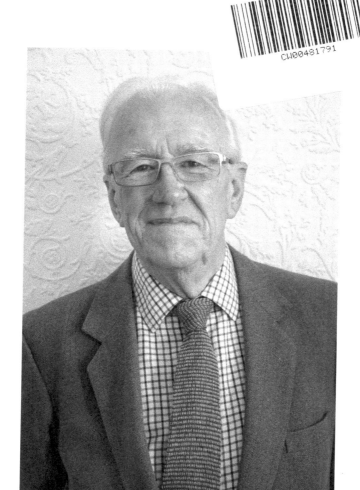

"Practice is not always perfect!"

This may hurt a little...

Acknowledgements:

Tom Bradshaw-Smith for his help

Photo by Olivia Kennaway

Illustrations by Jon-Paul McCarthy

Dedicated to Ann, with thanks

www.DrJeremyBooks.com
www.facebook.com/DrJeremyBooks
Twitter: @DrJeremyBooks

This may hurt a little...

The life and misadventures of a country doctor

Dr Jeremy Bradshaw-Smith

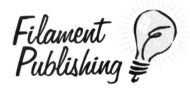

Published by
Filament Publishing Ltd
16, Croydon Road, Waddon, Croydon,
Surrey, CR0 4PA, United Kingdom
Telephone +44 (0)20 8688 2598
Fax +44 (0)20 7183 7186
info@filamentpublishing.com
www.filamentpublishing.com

ISBN - 978-1-910125-51-9

Printed by CPI Antony Rowe

Contents

In at the deep end   11

Early days   35

Progress   55

Partners   65

Standard days   69

Complaints and problems   81

Outside interests   91

Breaking and entering   103

Things that go wrong   111

Eccentrics and more   125

Night calls   137

Dying   151

Suicides   153

About the Author   159

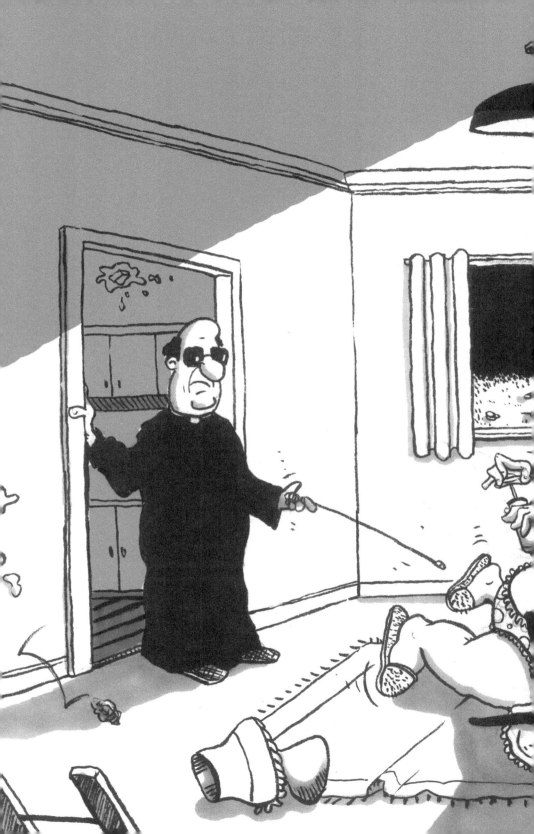

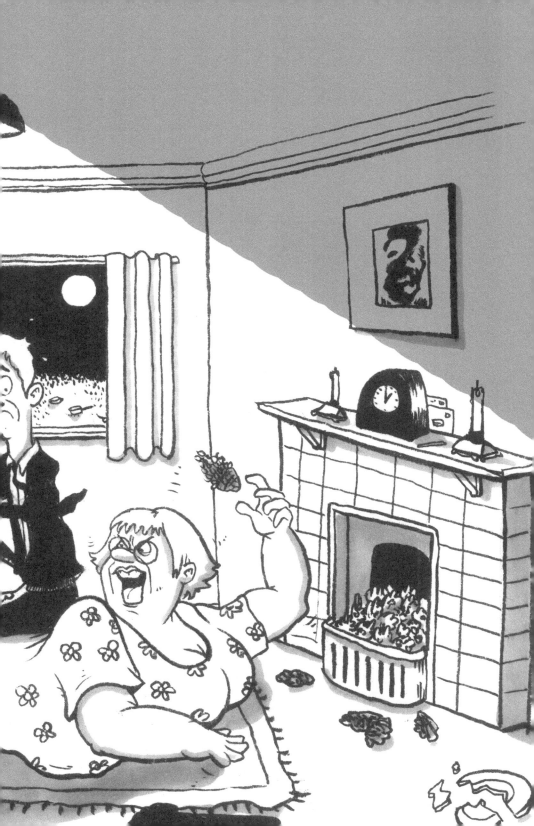

This may hurt a little...

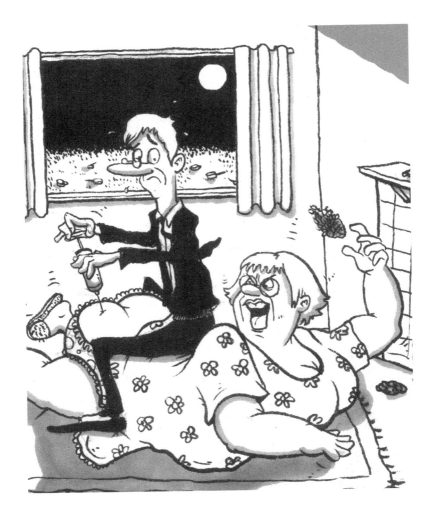

In at the deep end

If I had imagined that the first night call that I would make in my general practice career would have involved wrestling on the floor with a vicar's wife and pulling down her knickers, I would not have believed it could possibly happen. But it did.

It was 1964 and I had that day started on my thirty-year general practice partnership in a small country town. I had qualified as a doctor almost six years earlier and had worked in hospitals and had a short military episode before getting this job. National Service was still catching newly qualified doctors. After some two years as a hospital doctor I had foreseen my future career as a hospital physician. However whilst doing my military service I realised that looking after the soldiers and their families showed me that general practice was the kind of medicine that I wanted to do. It would give me the opportunity to get to know my patients and their families as friends and to become part of the life of a community. So after leaving the army I got a job as an obstetric house surgeon, in a first rate unit, with the object of getting a diploma as an obstetrician and so being well qualified in my role as a family doctor competent to deliver babies. I passed the necessary exams and was lucky enough to be offered a partnership in a well-regarded general practice, in Devon. This practice had its own small hospital and was allowed the use of the local large hospital's laboratories and X-ray facilities, a rarity in the NHS of the sixties. My contract with the NHS made me responsible for the patients on my list twenty four hours a day, for every day of the year. If I was away it was my responsibility to arrange and pay for locum cover.

The practice was a four man partnership at the time, and I was replacing a popular, hard-working seventy-four-year-old, one of the original founders of the practice. Another of the founding partners was coasting towards retirement. The next senior partner was the son of another original member, soon to take over as the senior partner. The fourth partner was a contemporary of mine and had joined the practice just four months before I did.

In the early 1920s three colleagues, fresh from service in the Royal Army Medical Corps during the First World War, had formed the first medical partnership in Devon and later, after the NHS had been formed, got together to build the first purpose built joint surgery in Devon; previously, as was then usual, the four partners had their surgeries in their individual houses. They were an innovative and far-sighted group of doctors.

My first day was bewildering; scores of strangers sat in a packed waiting room patiently awaiting their turn to be seen. Their medical records were held on small buff cards covered in by my predecessor's spidery "doctor's writing". When the card was full he would continue writing sideways down the card's edges, and then across the top and the bottom. Reading the previous medical history was somewhat like decoding a message and I had no Enigma machine to help. I got home at about 8.30pm that evening, exhausted but triumphant that I and the patients had survived.

In those days our long suffering wives managed the telephones when the surgery was shut. My wife Ann greeted me with the news that a local vicar had rung at 8.20pm, just before I got home, to say that his wife could not sleep and could the doctor call. A slightly strange request, she thought, at that time of day, but dutifully I picked up my bag and found my way to the Victorian vicarage in a neighbouring village. It was February and a pitch black evening as I walked up the short laurel wreathed drive towards the steeply gabled vicarage. I entered the tiny porch and rang the bell beside the stained glass mounted door. A shadowy figure appeared through the glass, the door was violently flung open and a female figure jumped out at me, arms raised and with a loud scream. My head must have almost hit the porch roof in terror.

It turned out that the poor woman suffered from manic depression and was in a hypomanic phase. To complicate the picture her husband was blind. She was cooperative with me and swallowed enough barbiturates to keep a prop forward asleep for a week. I saw her settled down and I went home for supper, and would sort out further care in the morning.

At 2.00am the phone went and a tremulous voice said, "She is awake." Astonished, I hurried back to the vicarage to find all hell had been let loose. There was a quarter pound of butter stuck to the kitchen ceiling, all the saucepans had been thrown into the frosty garden and most of the furniture was tumbled over. I decided to give her an intramuscular injection of paraldehyde, an unpleasant drug to use and to receive, but a highly efficient sedative, all that we had for these occasions before Valium came onto the market. To do this I had to get at her backside. The empty fireplace in their drawing room had a neat pile of large fir cones stacked in it and as I approached with the loaded syringe she was hurling these at me with great force and unerring aim. The English cricket team of that time had need of her. Her blind husband, poor chap, was huddled in a corner saying, "Oh dear, Oh dear" as the mayhem surged round him. I grappled with her, turning her on her face, sat on her back, pulled her knickers down, plunged the needle into her backside and order was restored. I turned her into the coma position and drew breath.

Her blind husband must have been terrified by the noise and the unseen chaos going on around him. I spent the next few minutes restoring some kind of order to the house, scraped the butter off the ceiling, and, armed with a torch, collected the saucepans out of the garden before going home to the comfort of bed with Ann, wondering if life here was always going to be so challenging.

The following morning she was admitted without a problem to the local psychiatric hospital to make a temporary recovery in the cycle of bipolar disease, all that was possible at that time.

National Service was still catching newly qualified doctors because their duty had been put off until they were qualified, though it had been stopped for the other eighteen-year-olds the year before I was called up. The army then trained me in tropical medicine which resulted in me getting the diploma in Tropical Medicine and Hygiene, which later, surprisingly, turned out to be useful several times in darkest Devon after returning from East Africa and leaving the army.

We had come back to England with our two Cockney-born children. They had accompanied us to Kenya, where the battalion, for which I was the Medical Officer, had been posted. At the time the Mau Mau uprising was nearly defeated. We found the country absolutely beautiful and the locals charming and blessed with a huge sense of the ridiculous. With independence on the way many European professionals were leaving and I was offered several doctoring jobs in Kenya, but tempting, though the offers were, we decided to return to England when my military service had ended.

General practice in 1964 was all reactive: patients arrived with a complaint and we did our best to diagnose the cause and attempt a cure. There was no proactive element in play; we chased clues as to what was going on, but did little to deal with problems that might occur in the future. Record keeping was merely primitive note keeping and consultant's letters were filed in the NHS small envelopes alongside the buff cards which held our handwritten notes. We were lucky in this area to have a consultant pathologist who liked GPs to use his laboratories and a radiologist who let us have access to X-rays. They rightly justified this because the local GPs were more accurate in asking for the appropriate tests than the newly qualified junior hospital doctors. This meant that, unlike many parts of Britain at that time, we could practice medicine in the way that we had been taught, using laboratories and X-rays to confirm or suggest the diagnoses. We also benefited by having a small hospital in our town, with a casualty and minor surgery facility, both of which were run by our practice. We also had the use of obstetric beds in another small town five miles away so we could take an active role in the management of our patients' labours and hospital deliveries.

The doctor that I took the practice over from had been a most dedicated man, and during the Second World War had worked all hours coping with all the difficulties thrown his way. He was seventy-four when I took over his practice and had been ill, so his previously high standards had slipped somewhat. I spent an afternoon with him in his car on his rounds the day before he retired. The first of his patients we called on was a nice old widower. "Hello, Coles," he greeted him, "haven't seen you for ages, this chap here is going to be your new doctor. He is a distant relation of mine so he will be alright." This was news to me! We spent some four hours on the road meeting several patients all of whom were reassured that one of his distant relatives would be their new doctor. At the end of the round we ended up at our original visit. "Hello Coles, haven't seen you for ages…."

When I called on Coles by myself a week or so later, Coles said, "Saying nothing against the Doctor, but I think it was time that he gave up."

My predecessor's wife would not allow him a television set so he used to spend his Saturday afternoons in a nearby village which housed some of his favourite patients. He watched different programmes in each of these houses; when the programme ended he would move on to the next house as rapidly as possible so as to miss as little of the next one as possible. Old Gertie would say with affection, "He comes through the door just after 'Dixon of Dock Green' has started, saying 'What's happened?' as he takes off his scarf." She then added, "And he dashes off at the end and often forgets to ask how I am." I went to his going away ceremony in the town's community hall where his patients had clubbed together and gave him, as a leaving present, a television set of his own.

When we negotiated the new practice agreement, we all agreed that if a partner wanted to continue in working in the practice after the age of sixty-five his share of the profit would reduce by one fifth for each subsequent year so that by the time he or she was seventy years old that doctor would be working for no financial benefit whatsoever. For our first three years as junior partners we only took a half share of the practice profit taken by the senior partners.

A delightful retired farm worker was being treated by him for heart failure and had been told that his heart was like a lump of jelly and that he would never leave his bed. In fact his problem, apart from old age, was a respiratory one and within a few weeks I had weaned him off his nightly morphine and he was well enough to be able to take an afternoon breather on his doorstep. I was thus lucky to have an initially easy run and have some successes which did my "street cred" no harm. In fact this old man became a talisman in my mind, like the ravens in the Tower of London, and as long as he lived I believed that all would be well with my practice.

Our small town was once an important market town with no major road going through it, which enhanced its ambience but diminished its importance. Fairfax and Cromwell had wintered their army in it during the Civil War and the lovely church still bore the scars of the vandalism of their occupation. By the time that I arrived in the town the cattle market had already ceased to function and three years after my arrival the railway line was taken up and the station closed. We still had our police station and Magistrates' Court, though a few years later they were also removed. The striking thing about the town was the welcome and the friendliness of the inhabitants. It was such a contrast to the ways of Londoners. The town was administered by our own Urban District Council which, eight years later, was swallowed up by a large district council. The small square in the middle of the town contained the more important shops including two garages with their petrol pumps still on the pavement, one of which had been a farrier's forge. A very narrow street led on up a steep hill to the magnificent church with its well-occupied churchyard, which was always beautifully looked after. Opposite the east end of the church a narrow gap between houses led to the little Victorian cottage hospital. The way into it was so narrow that it could only be used by the particularly narrow ambulances that the Health Service had to keep for the town.

The town still has several tiny little squares off some of the streets with clusters of small terraced houses surrounding an area the size of a netball court. Before sanitation came to the town this was where, mixed with straw, the square's inhabitants' nightsoil was stacked. The farmers would buy the dumps from the landlords to use as fertiliser and move it every few weeks. This was always a bone of contention with the square's tenants, who reckoned that as they had provided the material they should be the receivers of its bounty.

The mainstay of employment in the town was a factory that had grown up around a huge listed eighteenth century water mill that had once woven cloth. Over the years this had been transformed by the building alongside of factory sheds and when I came to the town it was designing and manufacturing high quality bespoke electrical switch gear. Over the years it changed hands more than once and eventually, when in the hands of an American company, it was shut. Currently it is empty, its development hampered by the listed status of the huge mill building. Once this had been closed, apart from a small engineering shop, all manufacturing in the town ceased.

Getting to know my patients was a joy. To a man and woman they were welcoming to both the new doctor and his family. An eccentric man wearing an old army greatcoat and army boots without socks became a regular sight. As he passed one in the street he would give a truncated salute and say, "Morning My Lord" or "Morning My Lady". My senior partners who lived in the town would come home to find that their garages had been immaculately cleaned by Herbie, and any donations given to him by them went to "the hospital". He lodged with a niece at her farm two miles out of town and would walk in daily to do his good works. As in most local long standing communities he was accepted, understood and enjoyed just as he was. Most of the local males in the town had a nickname which they had acquired at school and it stuck with them all their lives. There were several family names that were scattered about and numerous cousins, aunts, and uncles cropped up which made one aware that you were often likely to be talking to a relative of your last patient.

The first challenge in 1964 was that of getting a telephone. There was a waiting list of several weeks for ordinary customers of the Post Office to get a telephone line and an actual telephone. Often people were offered a party line which meant that if the other party was making a call when you wanted to telephone you could hear their conversation, so you put down the phone and tried again later. How you managed to share a line if both parties had teenage daughters I have no idea. In fact, as I was a doctor, it was recognised that my need for a private phone was unarguable and we were connected within two days and had the use of a single dedicated line.

There was no appointment system in use in the surgery, and patients were seen in the order that they arrived, some coming well in advance of the start of the surgery. The presence and murmur of a packed waiting room when one arrived to start the surgery could be daunting, and the pressure of knowing how long people had been waiting was always present. The patience shown by the public was heroic: the waiting, if you had not arrived early, could be monumental, and the wait, even for the early arrivals, was often considerable, sometimes reaching two hours.

Each of us was "on call" every night and weekend and all four of us covered each Bank Holiday and Christmas. This meant our wives were housebound every night and weekend. Having said that, most of our patients were very thoughtful, and a call early on a Monday morning was nearly always urgent, some people heroically putting up with a great deal of pain or discomfort so that their doctor could have a free weekend. With the NHS only having been in existence for seventeen years, the feeling that the doctor ought to be thanked still existed for some and our visits were often rewarded with a present of a cabbage or from farmhouses a jam jar full of clotted cream. Often a shallow pan of milk on the kitchen stove was seen processing that lovely cream. In those days nearly every farm had a milking herd and the milk churns on their stands at the farm gate were a familiar feature. Often one waited behind a herd on its way to the milking parlour. Good stockmen knew that hurrying the herd along reduced the milk yield and one learnt to be patient. With one herd the young man driving them could be seen with his arm over the back of his favourite cow who always chose to follow up behind with her favourite herdsman. Alas now only a very few of the local farms have a milking herd. Many of the large farmyards are now "barn converted" into housing as the small farms have been absorbed by the larger ones, leaving the old fashioned farm buildings too small for their contemporary purposes.

Home visiting was very much part of the day's work; often some fifteen to thirty visits were done in a day, so it was easy to get an understanding of the differing lifestyles of the different families. One winter a flu epidemic saw me seeing one hundred and eight patients on Boxing Day. This included the tragedy of a four-year-old boy drowning in a half empty swimming pool, his Christmas presents still under the Christmas tree. My last job late that evening was delivering a little baby boy which made me feel much better.

Percy had a small building business of which he was the boss and carpenter. He employed a bricklayer and a builder's labourer and they set a high standard. His firm operated beside his home, down an unpaved lane in a hamlet at the top of a hill. I got to know him because I looked after his wife, Phyllis, who suffered from very severe rheumatoid arthritis. Her knees had been so bad that to allow her to bear weight an orthopaedic surgeon some years before had fused both her knees, so that they were permanently straight. She had been converted into an old fashioned clothes-peg. This was some years before knee replacements had been made possible. She could work in the kitchen straddling a motor cycle saddle that Percy had converted for her to use. He was in the process of finishing off the job of building an architect designed luxury bungalow in the same lane when I got to know them. He was particularly delighted in being asked to put in a secret compartment in one of the rooms which, somewhat naively, he showed me with pride.

I asked him to build me a field gate for the end of my short drive which he was happy to do. Meanwhile Phyllis had a major flare-up of her arthritis and I had taken her in to the cottage hospital to be nursed until the flare-up had died down. I had seen the gate ready in his shed but it never appeared, so I asked him when it was going to be hung. "Not until you let Phyllis out of hospital," was his reply. Sure enough, the day after she came home the beautifully made gate arrived and was duly hung.

Sadly, when Selective Employment Tax was introduced, Percy decided that he could not afford to pay it and would go it alone. So rather than employing the two men he gave them notice and they were out of a job. Two shops in the town which employed drivers for their delivery vans also decided to dispense with the vans and deliveries and another two men lost their jobs.

Overweight patients would tell you that they did not eat enough to keep a robin alive, but a visit at a meal time would often show how robust a robin's appetite could be. A very few families lived in unbelievable squalor. One old widower had so much debris around in his cottage that you walked in a sort of trench system between door and fireplace and fireplace to kitchen. He had told his family that he had a treasure trove hidden amongst the mess in the house. When he died his family moved in as quick as a flash to clear the mess and find the treasure; they cleared the mess up beautifully, but, to their displeasure, found no treasure trove.

As junior partners we did our first three years' work on a half of the senior partners' share of the profit, which meant that my first year saw us two juniors earn about £800 each, not a princely return for long hours and responsible work. When we joined the partnership we also had to buy our share of the practice premises from the out-going partners which meant that we had to borrow the money to do so. To buy the quarter share of the surgery premises cost us new partners £1,000 each, which in 1964 was a great deal of money. After the three years our share of the profit reached parity and we could then afford a mortgage for our own homes. The banks regarded us as good risks in the future and the loans required were not difficult to get. Nowadays the new partners start on parity with their seniors, so the tough three years on half a share have gone. However, buying into the ownership of a share of the premises and equipment is still required. These costs are refunded to the retiring partners, after they leave, by the continuing and new partners. General Practitioners are self-employed subcontractors to the NHS and run their own businesses, but have to apply a certain quality of standards of their premises and what are deemed a proper number of surgeries to be done in the week. The problem was that any improvement to the service that we wanted to provide, such as secretarial help or employing a nurse, came out of our profits and cost us money. This showed up in the poor quality of infrastructure and ancillary help provided by some of the greedier practices.

As my probationary year was nearing its end, I was worried as none of the partners had mentioned that I was acceptable as a permanent partner. I eventually plucked up courage and asked our senior partner if I was alright, and could I be given a permanent partnership. "Haven't we mentioned it? Sorry, yes of course you are OK." A huge relief.

Our aged senior partner was persuaded to retire after I had been in situ for just over a year. The arrangement had been that he would go after I had been a partner for a year. However, though seventy six years old, he found life very pleasant, seeing perhaps only ten or so patients a day and drawing a full share of the profit. Our surgeries, when alongside his, were often interrupted by his smiling face coming around the door with a request to take blood from one of his patients as he could not manage to find a vein. The other junior partner was also doing most of his night work. After the year was up he told us that he might stay on longer as he was enjoying his life. It was gently pointed out to him that he was not pulling his weight and, like the gentleman that he was, he resigned from the partnership.

For the next five years we three remaining doctors ran the practice by ourselves, but new housing estates being built in the town and a nearby village had brought our numbers up to nearly nine thousand patients, a bigger list being the only way that one could boost the practice income, but cruelly hard work especially when a partner was ill or on holiday. We all called in on the hospital at least once every day of the week. On Sundays I would take the children with me and drop them off with Mrs Jasper in the hospital kitchen, where they would be spoilt, while I did my ward rounds.

Initially we were served by a single receptionist who knew the practice intimately and could usually find us by telephone, at a patient's house or a nearby shop, during our rounds when emergencies called. Unfortunately over the years she developed "the dragon at the gate syndrome" with the patients, and occasionally with one of us. Her end came when a most conscientious mother asked to know the dates when her child had been immunised. "You should remember," was her retort, "Yes, I know," was the reply. "But when we moved house I forgot where I had put the records." The rejoinder from our secretary doomed her. "I bet you did not forget to collect your family allowance," was her reply. As this had followed numerous other episodes of rudeness to patients as well as her once refusing to speak to one of the partners for several weeks, her removal from the scene was well deserved. She was soon replaced and from then on our ever increasing reception staff received nothing but praise; mark you, many of them had been on the receiving end of their predecessor's tongue and knew what it had felt like. One patient of a neighbouring practice told me that she had heard we sent all our receptionists to a charm school!

Our now senior partner was a man of generous spirit and once we two new boys were well established he asked us what changes we would like to see in the running of the practice. We both said that we would like to start an appointment system. "Would not work here," was the reply, "but if you two want it we will do it." Three weeks after it was implemented his comment was, "Brilliant, why on earth didn't I think of it?" Typical of him, an ideal colleague who never pulled rank, unlike some senior partners did in other practices.

We later started a rota with one night off a week, and after a time this became just one partner on call at night and weekend; harder work at the weekends, but blissful freedom to get dirty or drunk if one wanted to. It was especially good for our wives who were not continually tied to the telephone all weekend in case there was a call. An afternoon off during the week soon followed and then a whole day off, and the quality of family life was enhanced. None of this meant that we did less work, but concentrated it, and gave us time to unwind.

During my first weeks in the job I was continually under time pressure as I had to learn my way around the area that the practice covered, some fifty two square miles, and to get to grips with my patients and their needs and idiosyncrasies. This was most enjoyable, helped by our lovely countryside, but time consuming and my evening surgeries often stretched out until after 8.00pm. The rewards were that one felt that one was being useful and one's efforts were appreciated by the community.

One evening an elderly spinster, a Miss Pring, was the last patient in the long queue and produced a story that was so convoluted that in my mentally exhausted state that I decided to play for time. I suggested that it would be easiest if she stayed in her dressing gown the following morning and I would come round to her house to examine her. She was happy with this arrangement and I went home for a much needed supper and sleep. The following morning I arrived at the short drive to her house to find that the gate had two house names on it, one above the other, and the house down the short drive was a semi-detached one with no name on either entrance. I chose the first door and rang the bell. The door was opened by a familiar looking female, but not in a dressing gown. "Miss Pring?" I enquired. "Yes," was the reply. "I have come to examine you," I said. I was ushered in, gave her a thorough examination, found nothing untoward, reassured her and left.

Meanwhile in the next door house, the other sister, still in her dressing gown, was getting increasingly impatient and then irate. Later that day the Miss Pring who I had examined went round to her sister saying what a wonderful new doctor I was, going round all my elderly patients to examine them. This was not the view of the original Miss Pring.

Many years later the original Miss Pring was in the cottage hospital with a urinary infection and became very confused. One night the Night Sister rang to say that the old lady had climbed from the first floor window onto the sloping roof of an external corridor and had slid down it before she jumped to the ground unharmed and had run off unscathed into the night, clad only in her nightie. Night Sister said that she could have hit me when I asked, "Didn't you know that she was a trained parachutist?" To Sister's huge relief we found her before dawn in a lane nearby.

Once, halfway through a busy day, I was asked to see an elderly couple, who I was visiting regularly, as the husband was very ill with a terminal cancer. After they had retired from farming they had moved into a small Victorian villa on the edge of a nearby village. It had a nicely kept kitchen garden managed mainly by the wife. When this call came in from them for a visit it meant a five mile drive, which I managed to squeeze in between finishing the distant branch surgery and before going back to base for my evening surgery. When I arrived at their house they beamed at me and said that there was nothing new that was wrong with either of them but that they had wanted to reward me for the good care that I was providing. The old boy said, "Doctor, take 'ee this knife and go into the garden and cut any cabbage you like." Doctors were much appreciated and a "thank you" was common. Christmas time was always the season of presents to the doctors, and many patients gave us bottles of booze, turkeys and other very welcome gifts.

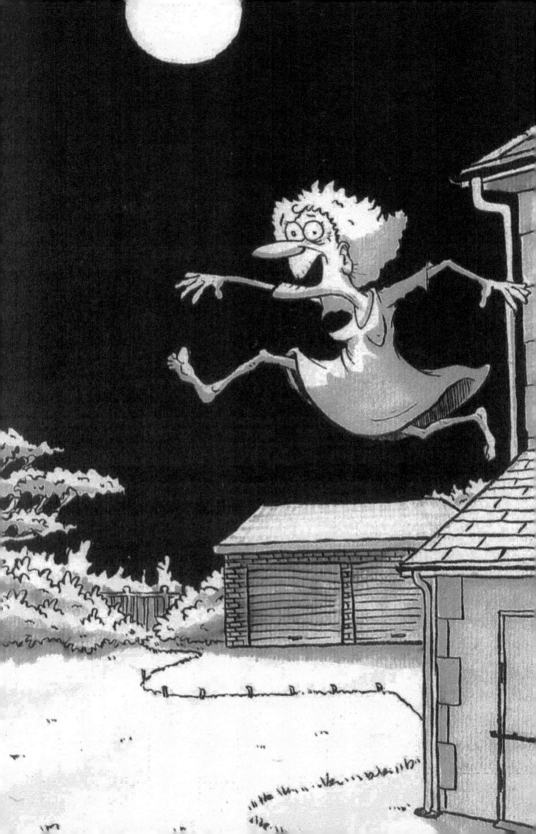

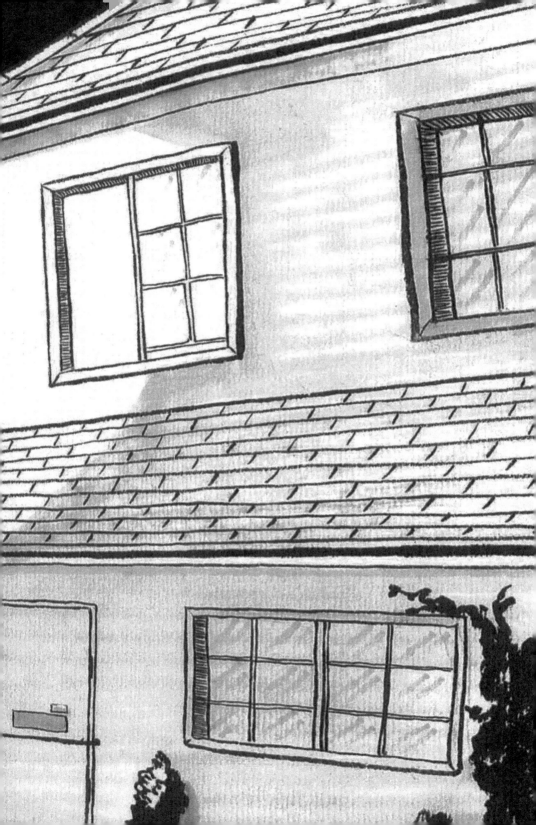

The same old man had a somewhat old fashioned view of marriage and the duties of a wife to her master. One morning when I was doing my weekly routine visit to him I noticed that, unlike his usual smartly turned out persona, he was unshaven. I asked if he was not feeling well as he was not his usual tidy self. "Tis urr," he replied, "Urr wouldn't shave me this morning." I found myself saying that he was such a miserable old bugger that probably with a razor in her hand she felt that she might not be able to stop herself cutting his throat. I immediately thought that I had gone too far this time, but to my intense relief, after a short pause, they both started laughing.

One could be caught out, however. I was looking after an old farmer in a lovely small Georgian farmhouse; their orchard was always ablaze with daffodils in the spring. He was suffering from Parkinson's disease. The house had no electricity supply and was bitterly cold. I suggested it would be better to keep more of the house warm, rather than having the kitchen as the only warm room in the house, because if he caught cold his difficulty in coughing, due to his illness, could lead to pneumonia. I suggested that it would be much easier to keep the house warm if they put in an electricity supply. The field next to the house was owned by the sick farmer's sister and was the only field in which the electricity board were prepared to put up the necessary pole. My patient's wife told me that his sister would not allow a pole to be put into the field, therefore there could be no electricity supply.

As it happened, that winter he did get ill with pneumonia. I took him into our cottage hospital where after a short illness he died. Very soon after his death I went round to have a chat with his widow. When I arrived and knocked, she opened the front door with the somewhat grimly truthful accusation, "Well, you did not save him." At the funeral, as the coffin was being lowered into the grave, with all sides of the family gathered round, the widow pointed into the grave and then at her sister-in-law across the other side of the grave and said, "He would not be down there but for you, and the doctor said so." Though untruthful, it was somewhat embarrassing, as I looked after both families. However the other family did not seem to hold a grudge about what I was supposed to have said.

The next summer she told me that she was fattening a goose for me for Christmas. For the next few months, progress on "my goose" was given whenever I saw her and I was thoroughly looking forwards to my present. Later she then told me that my goose was ready and to come round and collect it on Christmas Eve, which I did. She handed me the goose, plucked and drawn, with the words, "That will be ten pounds please, Doctor." One should not count one's geese before they are delivered.

Another surprise was meeting the then county coroner, a competent man with not a trace of pomposity and, as I discovered, a dedication for keeping costs down to a minimum. I had only been in the job for a few months when one evening I was called to the back of a shop because the owner had been found hanging from a beam there. There was a suicide note and the matter was straightforward. I wrote a written report for the coroner's officer and was asked to attend the inquest.

When I had to attend the Coroner's Courts in London, I was used to panelled rooms with witness boxes, the royal coat of arms displayed above the fine chair and desk at which coroners sat, and even a jury box for when the coroner decided that he needed a jury. Here there was a complete contrast. The inquest took place in a scruffy and bare back room in the local police station. There was a small rickety table at which sat the coroner, an austere (but in no way intimidating) man. Set out in front of his desk were four rows of folding chairs for the public; these were occupied by the numerous relatives of the dead man. I was asked by the coroner's officer to take my seat in the front row.

The proceedings started with the coroner saying, "Doctor, you are a busy man, so I will take your evidence first." He then continued that to avoid extra cost he would take my evidence as to the cause of death which had saved the cost of a post-mortem examination. I stood up and took the oath. I then, in response to his question, stated that in my opinion the victim had died from strangulation due to hanging by his neck from a rope tied to a beam. "Thank you, Doctor. I will give you your fee now and you can then leave the court to go about your business." He then wrote out a cheque and asked me to come forward to receive it. "That will save the cost of a stamp," he exclaimed with satisfaction, and I crawled out feeling somewhat embarrassed at the thought of being shown to take a fee for my part in the family tragedy.

Some strange beliefs were held by some people about death. I was called out one afternoon to a village hall, where the tea after a funeral service was being held, as one of the guests had collapsed. When I got there I found this ashen pale figure being held upright by two large men. I asked them to lower him to the floor where he quickly became a better colour and soon after was back to normal. He had had a faint in the stuffy, crowded room. When I asked the chaps who had been supporting the poor man why they were holding him up, I was told that it was common knowledge that nobody died when they were upright. Not a current medical view.

I could not visualise general practice without working for the National Health Service. Sending out bills to people who would have difficulty in paying must have been distressing and difficult to do. Both my grandfathers had been in general practice and had usually charged the better off patients more so as to subsidise the poorer patients. I had in all about twelve private patients, they wanted to be private in spite of being told by me that they would get the same opinion and the same treatment as if they were an NHS patient. The one difference would be that I would visit at their convenience, rather than expect them to come to the surgery if they were well enough to attend. In fact one of my private patients, a retired industrialist, would make his appointment and sit patiently in the waiting room with the NHS patients until called in turn. I once asked him why he bothered to be a private patient when he expected no privileges, to which he replied that he could afford it and thought that he ought to contribute more towards his health care.

Many years later, after I had given a lecture on keeping medical records on a computer at Duke University in the USA, I spent a morning with the nearest American equivalent of a general practice in Durham, North Carolina. It was a Tuesday morning and while standing behind the reception desk, I watched a plump motherly black woman approach and ask if she could see the doctor. The receptionist looked up her details and said that she owed the doctor fifteen dollars. The receptionist then reached across, and, without asking, took the woman's handbag from her, opened the wallet, extracted the only cash in it, twenty dollars, and handed the bag back saying that, yes, she could be seen. Being early on in the week, I assumed that was probably all the money that the poor woman had left until payday. I am grateful that we do not have that kind disincentive to receiving medical care in this country.

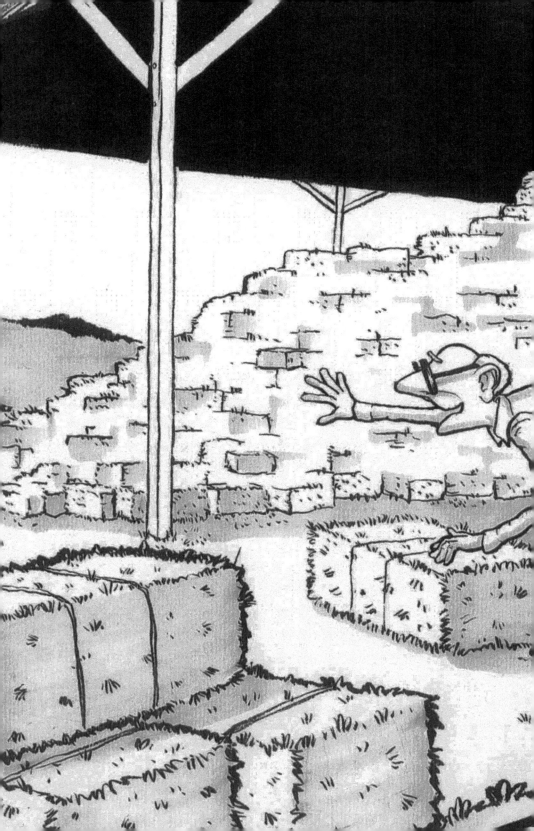

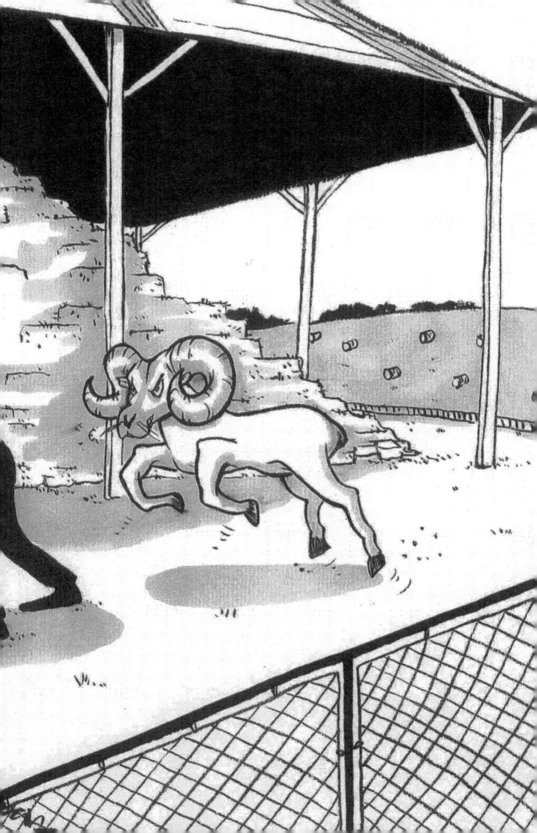

This may hurt a little...

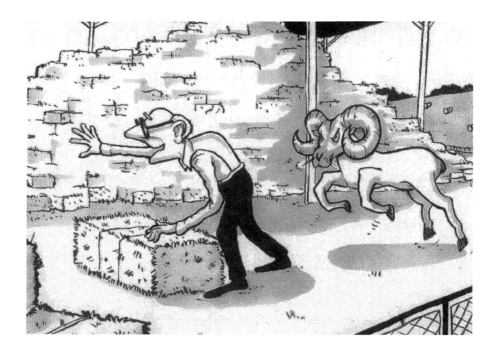

Early days

In the old fashioned way, within a few days of our arrival in the town we were called on at our rented house by all the butchers, grocers, garage owners and greengrocers, all vying for our custom. Of course we had no idea who would be the best choice, but Ann seemed to make the right decisions and we had excellent service from all her choices. There were four butchers slaughtering their own animals, four bakers all baking on their own premises and a wonderful hardware shop which held everything and anything that you could possibly need or want, sometimes at pre-war prices. The shop assistants were a contrasting pair. The male assistant was a giant of a man and his female counterpart as small a woman as you could possibly imagine. One of the four grocer's shops had a wonderful long mahogany counter and stated that "cheese is our speciality". Now we have only two butchers, one baker and no specialist grocer though a supermarket and a mini supermarket have taken the place of the lovely mahogany counter. The wonderful hardware shop, thankfully, still exists.

My first falling-out with one of the local tradesman was, as I saw it, an unavoidable shame. There were three local garages in the town, and I had fixed up for my car to be looked after by the easiest to get to and arranged to have an account with them. All went well, they did an excellent job and I could not have been more satisfied than I was with them. However, on one Saturday afternoon towards the end of my first winter in the town I was telephoned and asked to visit a man who had started vomiting blood. I went immediately to my old car and could not get it to start. I rang the garage that I used, who informed me that they could not help out as they were all going to a local family wedding. I then rang another of the garages who immediately said that their top mechanic was watching a local football match and that they would find him and get him along to sort it out.

Sure enough, in about half an hour the mechanic arrived, and handed me his car keys, so that I could get to the patient without delay using his car. By the time that I had sorted out the problem and got back home he was enjoying a cup of tea in the kitchen with my car mended and ready to go. He had missed the rest of the match and saved the situation. It then seemed churlish not to switch my custom to that garage which had been so very helpful, so I did just that. I later met my previous garage's owner in the street, who very aggressively accused me of a lack of loyalty. He was on my medical list at the time, but switched to another doctor in the practice, though his wife and sons stayed on my list.

We started living in a rented house in the middle of the town for six weeks, before being offered the tenancy of an ex-farmhouse, just outside the town, at the very reasonable rent of four guineas per week, on condition that during the first year of the tenancy I had the outside walls and window frames painted. There was no way that we could afford to pay a firm to do the job so I found an extremely friendly and competent man to help me with the task. He used to, on occasion, umpire some of our cricket matches. We set to on ladders with wire brushes in our hands to scrub the existing painted stucco walls before doing the painting. Hard work and nasty for the knuckles if one missed one's stroke. We had to take down the window shutters and found several sleeping bats hanging to the inside of them. The painting eventually got done and looked remarkably good and the landlord was delighted; I am not so sure about the bats.

After two years renting I made an offer to buy the house that we were living in, on next year's share of the practice profit. This offer was turned down by the owner, so we found a new, nearly completed house to buy with an acre of scrub around it which, bit by bit, we turned into a garden. We had a decent vegetable patch, and planted a small orchard in which we constructed a chicken run. On a summer evening after a busy day I found hoeing the vegetable garden extremely soothing and usually had one or more of the children to chat with as we worked.

The field alongside our new home was mostly used as pasture so we were flanked by either cows, bullocks or sheep. At that time much more hay than silage was made and when it came to collecting and carting the hay bales the field would be full of anyone that the farmer could find to help. One summer when the bales were nearly all collected, the farmer let his sheep back into the field, including a feisty ram. An old boy, who had been helping collect the bales, was bending over when the ram charged him and, targeting his backside perfectly, knocked him sprawling. It took several minutes before the general hilarity came to an end and work was resumed.

We needed help in establishing the garden, especially as the hedge bank between us and the road was totally untamed and was some fifteen feet wide. I elicited the help of a retired farm worker, Tom Board, who set about laying the one hundred and fifty yards of overgrown foliage into a hedge. Tom was a spare, tough man of few words but plenty of action. His flat cap was always in place and on the odd occasion when he took it off the contrast between his leathery face and his gleaming white pate was astonishing. He had been a hedge-laying champion and seemed pleased to be faced with the challenge. The hedge was trimmed, suitable long upright boughs were selected to be half cut through and bent to the horizontal and, if deemed necessary, were pegged down. This all took time and once a week he soldiered on until the whole length was laid and looked and stayed immaculate. The garden seemed to have doubled in size by the time that he had finished. He stayed on, coming once a week to help with the rest of the patch. He became more loquacious as time went by, once advising me to grow "highgeraniums" and to put lettuces under the flowering shrubs to save wasting growing space. When he dug our first crop of potatoes he divided up the harvest into two piles. The big spuds were called "gentlemen's potatoes" and the smaller ones were described as "them's pig's potatoes".

One day after I had driven him home he invited me into his home, with pride, to show me the huge array of presents given to him and his wife by their numerous children, grandchildren and great-grandchildren to celebrate their Golden Wedding. He was very much more talkative that day.

To get some lawn started I asked Mick Gillard to give a hand. Mick was a newly married self-employed gardener and handyman. The area next to the hedge at the front contained a vast tree stump. I asked Mick to reckon what it would cost to bury the stump, clear the patch and sow grass seed. I did not want an estimate, just a rough number to find out whether we could afford the cost. He gave me an idea of the kind of sum involved, was then told to go ahead and set out, hiring a digger and doing the job very nicely. When it came to the bill, it came to less than he had said that it might be. He told me that the digger had cost less than he thought it would. He grassed in another patch every year when we could afford it. Several years later I had the great pleasure of delivering his two children.

Tom Board aged, as we all do, and retired and I was managing the garden myself with difficulty. One evening as I was working on the vegetable patch the local roadman, George Bryant, climbed onto the hedge bank and suggested that I needed some help, and that he would be the man. The council was doing away with their length men, as they now had a headland plough that could do the job more quickly and cheaply, but not nearly as well as the men did. He continued helping me out once a week until he became unwell and another man of the soil, Charlie Virgin, took his place, having retired from the farm where he had worked for years. Charlie was a wonderful worker with hand tools but lethal with machinery. During his working life he had broken masses of machinery including turning over a tractor. His then boss saw it happen and said that Charlie came out totally unscathed, but ran away and hid when he noticed that the gaffer had seen it happen.

We kept Charlie away from the mower but he was terrific at digging out the remaining stumps and looking after the vegetables. He was devastated with the news when we told him, after all the children had left home, that we were downsizing, and selling the house, so we took an allotment in the town for his sake. We had moved into a barn conversion close to our old house with only a tiny garden and no room for a vegetable patch.

Ann had a marvellous char who was with us for years. Coming twice a week, Lily Lock was an old-fashioned cleaner; she had been trained in a "big house" and was thoroughly competent and hard working. She also babysat for us. She regarded babysitting as such easy money that unless she did something else as well, she felt guilty, so when we got back, unasked, she would have cleaned the windows, done some ironing, anything that she felt needed her input. She was a veritable jewel. Her only drawback was that when you said, "How are you, Mrs Lock?" she told you and went on telling you in great length and detail.

One morning on waking we could hear sheep close by and, looking out of the bedroom window, we saw a neighbouring farmer's flock of sheep filling the garden. They had breached his hedge three hundred yards away, crossed someone else's field, and were happily eating everything in the vegetable patch. I rang Oliver and said that his sheep had completely ruined the whole patch, and asked what he was going to do about it. "I'll tell ee what Doctor, you can go to any one of my fields and pull any turnip you like," was his reply. I responded that that would not do, and we settled on two loads of farmyard manure being put over the hedge for us.

We were happily ensconced there for twenty five years, until all the children had all left home. We then moved to the much smaller house with the much smaller garden, but still enough room to have the children and grandchildren to stay, though not all at once.

During our first year in the practice Ann had our third child. A couple of weeks before this event, our three-and-a-half-year-old son had climbed up the ladder behind me as I was painting the house. I heard him climb up and told him to get down at once, at which he jumped down. On landing he gave a horrendous scream; he had sustained a spiral fracture of his right femur. He was in hospital for two months and was still there when our third child was born. So at that time three of our then family of five were in hospital. This did not make for an easy life. To make things even more difficult, when the new babe was two weeks old he developed an obstruction of his large bowel and had to be admitted to Great Ormond Street Hospital. There he was nurtured for two and a half months before he was big enough to be operated on which, thankfully, completely solved the problem.

Thank goodness for a supportive wife who managed virtually single-handed in all ways, usually with great good humour, though once when I arrived late and with the supper ruined she remarked good-naturedly that she was obviously number 3,001 on my list of patients. Not far off the truth, as the family did come second to the practice a great deal of the time.

I was keeping a diary which gives an idea of the kind of days that one had and also the energy that we had available at the age of thirty four. Here is a three day quote from it.

Tuesday 30th January 1968 – "At times today I felt like giving up. I had an enormously rushed morning, after taking in a vast long morning surgery. This made me late for the branch surgery and I had a mad scramble to get round. The afternoon was more leisurely, but after the evening surgery I had to go to examine advanced First Aid for the St John's Ambulance Brigade. This took two and a quarter hours and was hard work. I failed two out of the sixteen candidates. They have an enthusiastic set up and deserve some help. Then I had a visit to do on the way home, finally getting back for supper at 10.15pm. We heard today that we will probably be allowed a fourth partner to take some of the strain. I sincerely hope so as there is an awful lot for the three of us to do. We will need larger premises I imagine. Total hours worked 12."

Wednesday 31st January 1968 – Another tough day having been out in the night at 4.45am to a delivery at the hospital and then had another delivery to deal with just as I was starting my ante-natal clinic. I was late getting in for lunch where I was grabbed by Tom Board who, fair enough, wanted to show me what he had done in the garden that morning. On to a branch surgery, for some solid work, which saw me getting home at 6.00pm. Later a consultant came round to do a domiciliary visit to a patient with me, had a drink with us afterwards and left. We had a couple of neighbours in to play Bridge after supper. Total hours worked 11."

Thursday 1st February 1968 – "Day off. Called at 3.00am to see Major Browne and heard the phone ringing as I got home, so straight out to the hospital to deliver a healthy baby boy. As I returned home I heard Ann on the phone and had to go out to see Major Browne again and finally got back to bed at 5.00am. Not much fun. Thank goodness it was my day off and the rest of the work was sorted out by 11.30am. Played squash in the afternoon. Fetched elder daughter from school and had time to chat to Mick Gillard who was building a fence for us. Four friends came to dinner and we did not get to bed until 12.45am. Total hours worked 5.5."

Whilst only I had to leave the bed, poor Ann had also had her sleep disturbed by the phone three times as well as by my returning to bed, and still managed to give a dinner party.

Not all patients were the reasonable people that the vast majority were. One Sunday during a flu epidemic I returned home from a series of visits to find that Ann was upset about a phone call that she had just taken. A grown man, whom I knew well from playing cricket and squash, was ill. His father had rung to ask for a visit to his flu-ridden son. Ann asked for his son's address and he refused to give it, saying that the doctor knew the address. Ann pointed out that I always wanted the address to avoid possible confusion. He still refused to give the address and then finished the conversation with the words, "Stop being stupid and do your job woman" and then slammed down the phone. I did happen to know the man's address so did the visit, which started with an unedifying row, as I berated him for being so stubborn and needlessly rude to Ann. Meanwhile the wretched flu-stricken son had to hear his father and doctor shouting at each other at the tops of their voices, before he was actually looked at. The result was a continued friendship with the patient but never an apology from his father for his gracelessness.

Before the mobile phone days and with few phones in private houses, before we got the radios in the cars, one was often out of touch with the surgery and at nights and weekends with one's home. The only time that Ann ever rang me up during surgery hours was when on an icy winter's afternoon she happened to turn her car over onto its side on a steep hill. No damage done to her, thank goodness, and not that much to the car.

Once when I was out all night with a woman in labour, because the midwife could not be found, her telephone being out of order, Ann brought round to the patient's house a bacon sandwich so that I could have a bite before starting the morning surgery. That evening, when I came through the door, she asked, "Who are you?"

Sometimes coming home down our short drive I would see a child's head looking anxiously out of the study window. This meant that a misdemeanour bad enough to warrant a father's input had been perpetrated. I had then to steel myself to do the heavy father act when I had been hoping to relax. I do recommend that doctors should marry nurses; they make wonderful wives.

GPs' children get used to the nuances of the parent's job and hopefully become used to the disappointment of promised outings, such as a trip to the cinema, being cancelled because dad gets home later than he promised. When our fourth child was seven years old I once heard her answer the phone at home and having listened to the caller she asked, "And how often are the pains coming?"

Before they started school I quite often took the two older children with me in the car for an afternoon of visiting rounds. This was fun for me and also nice for some of the chronically sick who enjoyed meeting the children, a bit of variety for the housebound patients in what could be a rather boring life. I also often travelled with our Springer spaniel bitch in the car, a companion for me and security for the car. After visiting families the children used to enjoy coming out to meet the dog, which the dog also enjoyed.

Whenever I parked outside a patient's house I always turned the car so as to face the direction that I was intending to go for the next visit. This was mainly so that I could make a quick getaway in the hope of avoiding one of the neighbours ambushing me with the words, "Normally I would not bother you, but since you are here, Doctor…"

After I had been in the practice some four years the excellent local Grammar School asked me to talk about sex to the class of twelve year old boys. A female doctor from the next door town was doing the same for the girls. Giving the lecture was a most interesting event. I had no idea how as a teacher one had a total oversight of the class and could see all the giggles, nudges and winks that went on during the talk. A diversion occurred when one of the boys fainted. I then realised how much my teachers must have known about what was going on and that they often they must have chosen not to pick up on it. In the class I recognised a boy who I looked after, and whose mother could, without turning a hair, be asked about the talk. Only about a week later I saw her in the town and said that I had seen her young son in the class when I was giving a sex talk and asked if he had mentioned it to her. "Yes," she answered. "He said, 'Mum, you'll never guess, Dr Jeremy gave us a sex talk today. Goodness I could have taught him a thing or two!'" I was never asked to repeat the performance.

I was looking after three elderly sisters and the husband of the eldest, who farmed on a smallholding in the back of beyond. The middle sister was suffering from Huntington's chorea, and was deteriorating remorselessly. I had no treatment to offer but used to look in every Sunday morning, mainly to help the morale of her dedicated sisters, and to let them know that they were not totally abandoned. I often used to bring the two eldest children, then five and four, with me for my benefit, if not theirs. The farmhouse was up a two hundred yard straight lane, and as one's car turned into the lane one got a view of the farmhouse back door at the top of the lane. I noticed that every time the car turned into the lane the old sheepdog, who was always laid down across the lane from the back door, would get to his feet and walk across the lane to sit by the back doorstep. I told the children that I had magic powers and composed a little dirge which I would sing as we approached the foot of the lane. "Oh dog…Do what I say dog…When I tell you… Move!" Getting the timing right was no problem and as I said "Move" the dog always got up and moved as instructed. For a short time the children were most impressed by their father's uncanny powers.

The sad follow-up for this family was that shortly after the death of the sister with Huntington's chorea her elder sister then told me about the problems that she had been enduring whilst totally committed to her sister's care. These turned out to be due to an ovarian cancer, which by the time I was told about it, was incurable, and she died less than a year later.

I once had only my eldest son with me in the car and had a routine visit to do for one of my few private patients, who was rather a snob. She was somewhat deaf, which, as it happened, turned out to be lucky. Before going into the house I had instructed my four-year-old son that, on the pain of severe admonishment, he was to behave impeccably. He sat on a small stool during the rather long consultation without putting a foot wrong. It must have been all too much because as we left he turned to his hostess and, using the worst word he could think of, said, "Goodbye Wee-Wee". I did not turn a hair until we got back in the car when I told him in no uncertain terms what I thought. He told me that he was fed up because she had kept saying how lovely he was. I hoped that with my unconcerned manner she would think that she had not heard correctly. This turned out to be a good guess as the next time I visited her, needless to say, without the offender, she volunteered, "What a charming well-mannered boy you have, Doctor. Breeding will out".

Later on when I had got to know my patients I would sometimes collect the more mobile chronically ill and take them with me on one of my afternoon rounds. They always spent quite a time sitting alone in the car, but at least they had a change of scene for a time and they seemed to enjoy the outings. We were able, during the round, to discuss their illnesses, what was planned and the future prognosis. The most interesting and useful passenger in this group was an old retired builder who lived alone, suffering from Parkinson's disease. As we toured the district he would inform me about the history of many of the newer houses that we passed. "I would not buy that one doctor, built in a rush, and the cavity walls full of mortar." "That one would be a good buy; it was built by the builder for his daughter with the greatest care." I am certain that getting to know your patients and, just as importantly, that they get to know you, is a vital ingredient to good general practice. If you are known to be on their side they are more likely to be on yours.

One day a forty-year-old spinster, whose parents had both died a few years before, came to see me in the surgery. I had seen quite a lot of her as she was a nice, but a sad and rather lonely person, who had genuine worries to deal with. This time, however, the consultation was totally different from our usual encounters. She told me that she was going to get married to a widower in a month's time and would like me to give her away at the church. I could not have been more pleased and flattered to accept and Ann and I had a lovely afternoon at the village wedding and reception.

There were few cars and fewer telephones about in 1964 and the local telephone exchange was housed in the ground floor room of a private house in a shopping street in the town. The excellent female telephonists could see the world go by whilst they plugged phone connections in and out. I was once trying to ring home from the surgery when the operator, recognising my voice, said, "If you are wishing to speak to your wife, Doctor, there is no point ringing, she has just walked by with her shopping basket"!

The night telephone calls were looked after by the house's owner who had a camp bed in the exchange at night. She did a wonderful job in what must often have been trying circumstances. One night she called me in the early hours saying that the person calling had asked for a particular partner to visit. As the person was a holiday maker and not a patient of that particular doctor, and because that doctor had been out the night before, she thought it fairer that she put the call through to me. A very fair decision, I agreed.

When our old patrician partner was persuaded to retire, we three remaining doctors decided to divide up his list between us geographically. I inherited a village with a branch surgery some three miles from our base. The surgery was in a small room at the front of a cottage with a paper-thin wall between it and the tiny waiting room. Fat Mary and her husband lived in the cottage where we rented the rooms, and I asked her to keep a radio on to help mask the voices during the consultation. She often forgot and on one occasion her bath above had overflowed, which made for a rather damp surgery. Consultations had to be held in low voices. I had a medical student with me one morning when a young, glamorous and rather histrionic female divorcee came in. At what seemed the top of her voice she exclaimed, "Doctor, you will never guess what happened to me last night. My ex-husband called in, tore off all my clothes and revelled in my naked body." The waiting room was totally silent and the student astonished.

On occasion during the early days an erring child would be brought in to see the doctor as a disciplinary measure. One was meant to point out the error of the child's ways to him or her. Not what we wanted to be used for and gradually this use of the general practitioner, to our general relief, died out. To my surprise towards the end of my career it was resurrected by a sixty-year-old woman bringing in her husband, apparently for that purpose. During a routine evening surgery I called the next patient, a man who was usually well, and that I rarely saw. He arrived accompanied by his wife of a similar age. No sooner had they entered the consulting room than the consultation started with her turning to her husband and saying in a demanding voice, "Go on, tell him." He started to say, "We had just bought a..."

when she broke in again with, "Go on, tell him". "A caravan," he continued. "Go on, tell him," she repeated. He continued, "When I was towing it home, I turned a corner too fast and it turned over and fell to pieces." "Go on, tell him," she repeated. "..and I had not insured it," he finished. "There," she said with satisfaction and they left the room, he presumably paid his penance.

One of the old doctor's patients, who I took over the care of, had been visited weekly by him. A retired farmer with intermittent heart failure, he was grossly overweight and the head of a farming dynasty in the area. He had fought in the Boer War with the Devon Yeomanry, and was a most engaging man to talk to. On our first meeting at 11.00am I noticed a bottle of whisky and two glasses laid out on the table. As I started the consultation he said, "You'll have your whisky now, Doctor." I declined at that hour and was from then on regarded as a somewhat wet young man.

Another very old man, living in lodgings in town, had also been in South Africa at the time of the Jameson Raid and had seen Kruger talking to the Boers on his stoep before the Boer War. He was in still in full possession of all his faculties and could recall the past wonderfully well. He had been declared too old to fight when he had volunteered to join up for the 1914-18 war. I took my elder son, when he was four years old, to meet him, so that he can say that he has talked to a man who was in his prime during the Boer War and when Queen Victoria was alive.

One of the joys of general practice was in getting to know a huge variety of human beings and their strengths and weaknesses. In this kind of practice one began to understand the family relationships; many of one's patients were cousins or otherwise related to each other, and in time, knowing the ramifications, likes and dislikes, helped piece together the social structure that made the community tick. As the years went by the number of houses grew and with that the population expanded. I always felt that I was lucky to have inherited a list of locally born characters steeped in the ethos of the town as most of the incomers went onto the lists of the newer doctors.

The continuity of care was also very rewarding. Towards the end of my thirty years in the practice I delivered a young woman of a baby girl. After every delivery I was in the habit of placing the new arrival on the mother's tummy and examining the naked new-born child in full view of the parents. I commented to her that the baby "had all her fingers and toes." She laughed and said "Mum told me that that was what you said when I was born!" I had not changed the script in all those years.

Early on I was called to see old Tom Wilson, a former farmworker. Though now in his late eighties his huge hands and strong forearms still gave the impression of great strength and endurance. He was long since widowed, but he and his wife had bought their cottage in 1926 for £30 and lived there ever since. He had fallen out with his boss about Lloyd-George's stamp, had refused to pay it and therefore had no pension. He lived off his immaculately planted walled kitchen garden and on less than £2.00 per week from savings, invested in a strange London bank, on which he was paying tax. He spoke unaffectedly in the Devon vernacular. He would talk of "a girt great rank of tatties", a cough was "tissicky", twilight "dimpsy", roots were "mores" and being confused was "mazed" and, above all, the word for feeling on top form was "viddy". It is increasingly rare nowadays to hear some of those words used by the locals.

He asked me to call to see him. When I arrived, he started the conversation with, "Youm be a clever young man and I will give you ten pound if you can cure my itchy arse." I assured him that I would do it for free and had a look. I prescribed what was appropriate and returned a week later to check on him. "Youm be a clever young man, you have…almost cured it," he told me.

Three years later he decided that he was dying and I was called again. He had his long-standing farming great friend with him. After examining him I assured him that he was not dying and was good for a bit longer, when he blurted out that he had cheated me out of ten pounds because in truth I had cured his "itchy arse". I said that I had realised that and anyway I was not allowed to accept money for treating people. His friend chipped in, begging me to take the money. He said that Tom had harped on and on about it for the last three years, saying how much it was on his conscience that he had cheated the doctor when he had actually been cured. Under that pressure I took his ten pounds. I had by then re-organised his finances, doubling his income, and had got his overpaid taxes back, so did not feel quite so bad about it. At that time I had just lost my fountain pen so with the money bought another, which I still have. He lived for another two years and died with a clear conscience.

Wart charming produced an interesting conundrum. I was told that there were three wart charmers in the area, two of whom I knew. The charmer in our most distant village, whose identity I never discovered, was also said to be a dab hand with ringworms. The kerion is a large pustular ringworm coming from contact with infected cattle, it is never seen in town dwellers, and has now become a rarity in our local countryside. The wart charmer in the town had a following and my research into his success rate showed that though he had a less than one hundred percentage cure rate, he had several triumphs on record. However in one of the council houses in another nearby village was an elderly widow who excelled in this strange power over the common wart.

My senior partner told me that she had cured one of his son's warts and recommended her as a standby cure. Our younger son had a particularly enduring wart on his hand when he was eleven years old, which had survived all the usual removal methods, cutting out, freezing, silver nitrate stick treatment etc. Finally I suggested to him that he should see her. I gave him her address and he rode off on his bicycle to see her. When he came back I eagerly interrogated him on what she had done. "Nothing," was his reply. He had knocked on her door and when she answered it she said, "I suppose you have come about a wart." He replied that was indeed why he was here. She then asked his name and said to him that he was not to say "Thank you" and that the wart would go in a few days. She did not touch him or the wart. To our surprise and delight it vanished and never returned.

The common wart is a virus infection that in time, as with other viruses, the body builds up an immunity to, and they do vanish. Presumably this "charming" enhances the body's resistance and swats the wart more quickly, but how and why?

Having had this very effective demonstration I used to refer patients with persistent warts to this charmer. One recently arrived patient had some fifty warts all over her hands and I suggested that she called on the charmer and I forgot about it. A few days later I was in the town square when my patient came out of the butcher's, dodging through the traffic, shouting, "They've all gone", while thrusting her hands out towards me. The square was far from empty and it was a second or two before I realised that she was referring to her warts. Indeed all the warts had gone.

We had a tragedy on our hands when a well-regarded local tradesman strangled his wife. She was being repeatedly unfaithful to him and so they argued a lot, but he had never been violent to her. One day during an argument about her repeated infidelity she told him that she was going to leave him. They had two sweet little blonde daughters of two and three whom he adored. She told him that she would take the little girls with her and she would be nasty to them just to hurt him. His self-control snapped and he put his hands around her neck, squeezed, and she died. He then took the small girls to his mother's house, asked her to look after them and then went to the Police Station and reported to them what he had done. He was arrested and charged with murder. At his trial various witnesses, including a local JP, spoke on his behalf and he was found not guilty of murder, but guilty of manslaughter, and sentenced to a few years in prison. He served his time with full remission for good behaviour and came home to his village, his job and his daughters. He married, a very nice supportive woman, and family life resumed.

A few years later, while his daughters were still at primary school, a drama occurred. The teacher had noticed some bruising on the neck of one of the girls. On that Friday evening the school teacher rang the police giving a garbled message which was interpreted as "that a man had murdered his wife and was setting about one of his children". A police car raced to their address and the police burst into the house to find the little family around the kitchen table peacefully enjoying their tea. The experienced female inspector present realised that the situation was quite different from that reported, and saw that there was indeed bruising on the neck of one of the girls. There were finger bruises on the back of her neck and two thumb marks on either side of her lower lip. The explanation given fitted the bruising perfectly. The night before during tea she had stuffed her mouth far too full and started choking. Dad had grabbed her head from in front and with his two thumbs forced open her mouth whilst her step-mum had scooped the food out with her index finger and no harm was done. The inspector was perfectly happy that nothing criminal had happened, apologised and left the house, and tea was resumed.

It did not end there, however. Social Services became aware of the event and on Monday morning I was telephoned by a male social worker. He had not seen the child or family or talked to the police, but made a decision that a Place of Safety Order be placed on the child and that she should be taken into care. I persuaded him to allow the girl to be admitted to hospital instead of being taken into care. This struck me as a much more acceptable arrangement for the neighbours to gossip about. A very humane and understanding consultant paediatrician, on hearing the story, agreed to admit her to one of his beds at the district hospital that afternoon.

The Social worker issued the Place of Safety Order the following day in the hospital ward when seeing the child for the first time. By now the consultant, the GP and an experienced police inspector had all agreed that the bruising was consistent with the story from the parents and that the child had come to no harm or risk of harm. The social workers were adamant that the Place of Safety Order would stay on in spite of the evidence that it was an error. I asked the child psychiatrist consultant to examine the girl. After seeing her, his view was that she was likely to suffer psychological damage being kept in hospital away from her family. My paediatric colleague wanted the bed that she was occupying back. A meeting with we three medics who were involved, plus the police inspector, was arranged with the social worker and the deputy head of Social Services. At this meeting the social services refused to withdraw the Place of Safety Order but would "allow it to lapse", and the girl went happily home. I can accept that errors of judgement occur, but to take this kind of action without seeing the child or family before making a judgement is totally unacceptable.

I have twice been bitten by dogs during my rounds, once with no blame attached to the dog. I had walked in through the front door of a house that I was familiar with, without knocking. This so surprised the old dog asleep in the hall, that he bit me on my ankle as a reflex action. Not his or the owner's fault, and only a minor wound. The other dog that got me was a large Chesapeake Bay Retriever. This dog had previous form and only a week before I had sewn up a nasty triangular flap wound on the wrist of the milkman which had been inflicted by the same dog. I had been asked to visit a sick daughter at this house. I was just getting out of the car when the dog, loose in their drive, got me by the right shoulder, tearing the tweed of my coat as well as tearing the skin of my shoulder. My shoulder would heal but the coat was a more difficult challenge. The suitably apologetic owners paid for a very good invisible mend to be performed on the coat and all was well.

Going into a pub one evening to see the publican's feverish young daughter gave me a scare. I went in via the back door which was my usual way when entering pubs in the call of duty. As I walked in I found myself, to my horror, gazing eye-to-eye at a large bull mastiff, only a couple of yards away. He came almost up to my shoulder. To my relief he did not seem to mind my sudden entry and escorted me to his owner.

Progress

After a couple of years in the practice, the county council asked us if we would sell them our present surgery, so that they could build on to it and turn it into the first Health Centre in Devon. This purpose built surgery, that we had had to borrow to buy into, had been the first central surgery in Devon. It had been built by the previous partners who up till then had each been practising from their own homes. This building was comprised solely of an office, waiting room and the only two consulting rooms with their two examination rooms.

Keen to pay off the debt incurred in buying our share of the premises, we agreed to the sale and from then on paid a rent for the bit of the building that we used, and were repaid the rent by the NHS for doing so. However in time, as the population around increased and as more partners joined the practice, we needed to expand the building. The county council could not afford to do this for us. We gave up on the Health Centre and went into debt again to buy land and build our own much larger and more convenient surgery in a different location. There were five of us in the partnership by then and the luxury of not having to share a consulting room was wonderful. Previously, if one's surgery was running late, the knowledge that another doctor was champing at the bit to start his surgery was not conducive to good practice.

One day an Australian doctor arrived to see our set up. He had been sent by his government to investigate general practice in the British National Health Service. He had asked at the Ministry of Health where he could find the best general practices and was told to come down to the West Country where the uniform standard was excellent. When he asked the Devon powers that be the same question, they sent him to see us.

We had developed a reputation for being an innovative practice and in 1969 it was suggested that we might like to cooperate in a morbidity survey, financed by the government. An earlier survey had been carried out in a nearby city, but the sheer volume of the data accumulated on paper had been hard to analyse, so it was suggested that the next survey be done using a computer, at that time a daring concept. The initial idea was that we should write a second record at the time of the consultation, the diagnoses from which would be coded by trained assistants and then stored in a computer, which would then be able to sort and analyse the results. In those days the capacity for the storage of data on a computer was the limiting factor, so squeezing the physical volume of the data was always aimed for, hence the need for coding.

We agreed to cooperate with this scheme, but on our terms, which were starkly different. I had been given the task of researching into this and had found out that all the previous attempts at computerising medical records had failed. This was because busy doctors always got behind in writing up the duplicate record, and then never caught up. Secondly, validation of the accuracy of the coded data should always be done by the originator of the data, and no busy doctor was going to plough through the codes interpreting the diagnoses to check that the coding was correct. We said that if we were to cooperate we would want to write our notes in what passes for medical English onto a computer at the time of the consultation and using our own words. This would be the only record of the consultation that we would make. The computer jargon of the day was called "Real Time". Theoretically we would be a "paperless" practice and the first in the world to do this for every patient on our books. Do not believe a word of it – "paperless", indeed! We found that we used a great deal of computer paper. Thus serendipitously the keeping of general practice records on a computer was pioneered.

These terms were agreed and a superb team of computer experts were recruited and the design of the system went forward. All this was paid for by the Ministry of Health. Another part of this same team was also designing records for hospital use and for public health use. As the GP designers we met on most Monday evenings for two hours with the two Systems Analysts and on occasions any other doctor who wanted to have a say in the designing of a computerised medical record could attend, however only one other doctor ever joined us and then for only one session. The Systems Analysts made it clear that we were the experts on medical record keeping and what we wanted in the record, whilst they knew about computing and how they wanted to do it. However what we wanted in the record was paramount, and they would do their very best to provide it, which they did. It was a very happy and cohesive partnership.

A large air conditioned building was constructed in the district hospital's grounds in a town eleven miles away and a data line connected us to it. At that time a GPO engineer said to me that he pitied us as none of them knew anything about data lines. During the Queen's Silver Jubilee celebrations a string of coloured lights was inadvertently strung around the data line which caused interesting problems with the computer data transmission. Inside this new building was a mass of equipment, several washing machine-sized disc drives, four coffin-sized processors and a line of broom cupboard-like cabinets reeling out tape to the accompaniment of flashing lights. It was then space age stuff and now "x" times the computing power is contained in a Blackberry. A team from the USA arrived to see the set-up on a day when the air conditioning had failed and apparently were enchanted that some electric kettles boiling away in the computer room was an adequate substitute.

It was five years in gestation and towards the end of the process we had started to summarise our existing paper records, no mean task. I averaged six minutes to summarise each record and aimed to do ten every day. The task took nearly a full year to complete, as there were at that time some three thousand records or so for me to do. Sometimes if one was lucky the ten records were slim and took no time and little effort to summarise, but on unlucky days they were fat records that took ages to sort out.

We were ready to go in 1975, and started using the computer for our record keeping. In the November of that year we were the first practice in the world to print prescriptions. The negotiations with the ministry to allow this improvement were Byzantine. The local chemists must have been delighted to have legible scripts to decipher. We sat with these enormous grey Visual Display Units on trolleys at right angles to our desks, so placed that we could sit on swivel chairs knee-to-knee with our patients and swing round to enter the record on the VDU. On the lower shelf of the trolley was a printer loaded with blank prescription paper. The presence of all this kit made no difference to the nature of the consultations, though to start with most of our clientele showed some curiosity but no hostility to the set-up. Turning to make an entry in the record would stop conversation, but then picking up a pen to make a note had had the same effect.

The British Computer Society later gave the project an award for the computing most beneficial to mankind. This was a very welcome reward for the great deal of extra work which we had all put in, not least the excellent computer team. When I retired the team gave me the award as a very much appreciated leaving present.

In 1976 I had a paper published in the British Medical Journal describing what we were doing, which resulted in my being asked to read a paper on the subject of modern medical record keeping, and how we were doing it, at an international Medical Computing Conference in Berlin. My talk was delivered in English and simultaneously translated into French and German.

I made my usual rather weak joke about the only confidential feature of the traditional record being that nobody could read the doctor's handwriting. There was immediate laughter from the English speaking part of the audience, followed a second or two later by the French and Germans when they heard the translation, a somewhat unexpected happening.

We had spent a long time on discussing the question of the confidentiality of computer records, knowing how important, and rightly so, the secrecy of a medical record is regarded by one's patients. This was long before the Data Protection Act and we were pioneering in this field. We tied it up so tightly that we could even not allow another of our partners to view a particular record, or a part thereof, if that was what a patient wanted, though in my whole time in practice only one patient asked me to do that.

We backed up our records in the surgery every evening and also produced microfiche copies of the records which we kept, with a microfiche reader, in our cars. Later on, after they were produced, we carried laptops to the branch surgeries so that we could have complete and updatable records in all the branch surgeries and be connected to the surgery computer.

A few years later at a meeting with the BMA, on the ethics of computerised medical records, it was agreed that patients should be entitled to see and have a copy of their record, but should pay the doctor ten pounds to compensate for the trouble and cost of producing the copy of their record for the patient. I came back from London enthused by the idea. By then we had spent hours summarising the records of some twelve thousand patients and as a compensation for the time spent, as a money spinner, it was too tempting to miss. We organised some publicity handouts, suggesting that our patients should hold a copy of their records. These were duly distributed and we waited for the money to roll in. Alas only one patient availed himself of the offer!

I also spoke about computerised medical records to numerous medical gatherings in this country and at Duke University in the USA, and a partner lectured on the subject in Australia. Our practice was visited by doctors from all over the world to see this technological marvel, nowadays a very matter of fact feature on doctors' desks worldwide, but then a very dubious experiment. Many of the questions asked after my lectures were extremely hostile, as if we were somehow befouling general practice. At one lecture a doctor turned up wearing a space helmet and getting a good laugh.

I was once sharing a platform with an admirable GP from the Forest of Dean who had created a punch card index for his practice which represented a great deal of hard and useful work. He could manage the practice well but had had to forecast what he thought that he would need to know in the future when constructing his index, whereas we could interrogate anything that we had included as we updated the record. When the question time came most of the questions came to me, because what we were doing was such a novelty. He suddenly burst out saying that the women he employed were the best in his area, implying that those using computers were lesser mortals. I was able to reassure him that our employees were also the cream of the town.

We had polled our patients to see if any of them would mind their records being kept on a computer. Only one family objected; the father had been made redundant when a computer was introduced to the firm that he worked for, an understandable point of view for him. Anxieties that patients would recoil from the screens were groundless, and a patient of mine once came back from a holiday away during which he had needed to see a doctor, saying they were really out of date there, no "tele by the desk", not realising that we were the only people in the world at that time doing what we did "with a tele by the desk".

A major benefit of the computer record was the ability to interrogate the patients' records. We could find out how many of our patients suffered from specific illnesses. The first search that we did was within days of "going live". A report came in of possible side effect of a drug then commonly used to control blood pressure. Within twenty minutes we had a list with names, addresses and telephone numbers of all our patients taking that drug. It was then easy to recall them and deal appropriately with the problem. We could now plan to identify and recall people with the likelihood of having ongoing medical problems, taking a more proactive approach than was possible with the traditional records. Our computer could search for things that we had no idea that in the future we would want to know. For instance one of our partners always added an extra 'l' to the name of an antibiotic. We all knew that he made this spelling mistake, so that when searching for the use of that particular drug we could also search for the name with the spelling mistake of the extra 'l' in it.

Another benefit was the ease of finding a cohort of people with a particular diagnosis or problem and reviewing them. Our first target was a group of patients who had previously had either a partial thyroidectomy or treatment with radio-iodine (I131) as a treatment for an overactive thyroid gland. The symptoms of an underactive thyroid gland come on gradually as a sometimes late side effect of these treatments and are often regarded by the sufferer as due to "getting old". We picked up several patients with this condition before they realised that they were ill and going to get worse. It was most rewarding.

Altogether the ability to get pro-active management, monitor compliance with treatment regimes, and keep routine immunisations and services such as cervical cytology up to date was rewarding. The chore of not handwriting repeat prescriptions and the automatic logging of their provision was another massive benefit, appreciated by both us and the pharmacists who now could easily interpret the scripts.

I was once or twice confounded by believing what the drug prescription record showed about the patient's compliance with their drug taking. On one occasion a, supposedly intelligent, widow had a dangerously high blood pressure that I was attempting to treat with an antihypertensive drug. After an initial slight improvement in her blood pressure level, after some time the blood pressure stubbornly refused to get down to a safe level. I checked her medication screen, which showed that her pills had been asked for at the correct timings, which indicated to me that she was complying with the treatment regime. I increased the dose bit by bit with absolutely no improvement to her blood pressure. I eventually admitted to her that I was really worried that even on this very high dose of the drug I was unable to control her blood pressure and if we did not succeed in reducing it she might well have a stroke.

The following day I was called to her house by her friend who said that my patient had passed out and was still flat on the floor after getting up for breakfast. I rushed round to their house to find her conscious but every time that she tried to get up she fainted again. She had not had the threatened stroke. On checking her blood pressure I found it barely recordable. What I then discovered was that though she was ordering her blood pressure pills at the correct times she had actually not been taking any of them. When, the day before, I had mentioned the possible consequences of the continued raised blood pressure at that high a level she got a fright and had started to take the pills but at the very high dosage that I had ended up prescribing. This was of course much too high a dose and when she did take that dose her blood pressure dropped to virtually zero. We both learnt a lesson that day.

Another bulky woman with a slightly raised blood pressure was also diligently ordering the mild drug I was using in an effort to control her blood pressure. She had lost a little weight and her blood pressure came down somewhat though it was not ideal. I decided to maintain her at that level and she continued to get her prescriptions on the due dates. She died a couple of years later from a different cause. Shortly after the funeral her daughter-in-law telephoned to ask me what she should do with all the unopened packets of blood pressure pills that she had found while turning out the old ladies chest of drawers. Yes, she had always ordered on the due date, but had never taken any of the pills.

As we got familiar with using the computer system we started to design what I called control screens. Graphically recording the drug dosage alongside the test performance for patients on anticoagulants was easy enough. It got more complicated when designing screens for monitoring more complex diseases such as high blood pressure and diabetes, but these screens were gradually brought into use. The other value of these screens was that by following the agreed protocols they were often more accurately completed by the practice nurses, who we were now employing, than the doctors.

After a few years the relevant computer machinery had got a somewhat smaller so a small room at the surgery was air conditioned and used to house it. All it needed to contain was a washing machine sized disc holder, a broom cupboard sized processor and a large printer. The problematic data line was thankfully no longer needed. Our staff coped with the backing up of the records, booting up, and switching off the machinery, proving that ordinary mortals could cope with the mysterious world of the computer. Later of course air conditioning became unnecessary and the whole storage and processor were accommodated in the familiar small tower. The large original building in the neighbouring town is now used as the local ambulance headquarters.

We were paid by the government for our time and effort with the computer and used that money to install a portable radio system in our cars, one of the sets of which could also be taken into the houses of the duty doctors. Our wives thus also became radio operators. This was a godsend, saving us retracing our steps when a new call came in, and also in getting calls from our wives at the weekends asking if we could pick up a loaf of bread when on the way home.

One night I was called after midnight to see a child with earache and while on the way back home from their village my wife called me over the radio to say that a diabetic patient was in an insulin coma in the town. Just before I got to the house she called again to say that a known epileptic sufferer was having a series of fits in a house one hundred yards further on. I arrived at the diabetic's house, found the patient in his bedroom and was giving him the intravenous dextrose that he needed before his wife got back from the public telephone. When she did get back she went quite pale at the shock of finding me there already. I then drove to the epileptic's house, sorted that out, called in on the diabetic on the way home to check that all was still well and went back to bed, an hour's work in one go when previously I would have been in and out of my bed and the house three times. Now of course with mobile phones such technology is out of date, but at that time it was very valuable.

Partners

As the patient numbers increased it became necessary to increase the number of doctors. Our policy was that all new doctors would come in as full partners though only on a half share of the senior partners' reward for their first three years. If at any time during their first year they were not happy the new partners could opt out or the existing partners could decide that the new recruit did not suit. In fact that eventuality never occurred. This meant that at the partners' management meetings the decisions made had an input from all the doctors working here. At meetings we always came to a consensus view and never had to vote. Every time we chose a new partner we worried that the pleasant cohesion that we all enjoyed would be disrupted but luckily that never happened. The three partners that we started with became seven over the thirty years that I was there. Nowadays new partners come in on an equal share of the profit and there are several half-time partners which can produce problems for the patients and the management of decision making in the practice.

Because of the example set by our original senior partner, the new doctors had equal rights, if not equal incomes, as the existing partners. We always chose our holiday dates in rotation; the first to choose one year would be the last to choose the next year, and so on. We also always gave any new doctor time off for his first Christmas in the practice, feeling that they might like to have family to stay with them, and to see their new setup. Bank Holidays were shared out equally in rotation so there could be no feeling of injustice about it. We always wanted the partner, male or female, to be married, with a family or one in prospect, on the grounds that until you have heard your own baby crying all night you have little understanding of the stress that it causes.

Choosing the new partners in the early days was pretty informal. We would hear that someone was on the search for a job, ask them down, show them around and if we all liked them, offer them the partnership. Later when we already had five partners and our much admired senior partner decided to retire we advertised in the medical press and had over one hundred applications for the job. Some of these came as scruffy, unappealing, stencilled and formatted letters with blank sections where the name of the town was added and so on. Others were well-presented, computer-generated CVs. Shortlisting was done and some eight prospective candidates were invited, at their own expense, to spend a weekend day with us which included their spouses. Each of us had a segment of the practice to show them, the surgery, hospital, computer, branch surgeries and the practice area. Three of us would also give them and their wives coffee, lunch and tea. It must have been very stressful for them and it was certainly hard work for us and our wives, whose views were also sought. Once they had all been seen we would meet to discuss the candidates and come to a consensus on who would fit in the best.

We each tried to have a special medical interest; one partner was a member of the Society of Manipulative Medicine, one of us had the MRCP, and another partner was interested in dermatology, one an obstetrician and so on. Thus we could, if we thought it appropriate, refer diagnostic problems or patients requiring a different skill to a more practised partner.

We had the most difficulty when we were trying to find our first female partner. We realised that a female doctor's presence was needed, but to find a full-time married female doctor in those early days was not easy as, unlike today, not very many female medics were being trained. This was due to a considered policy in the medical schools that training women in medicine was not a good use of an expensive resource, as they were unlikely to continue in full-time practice. However we eventually succeeded in finding an excellent married female doctor who more than pulled her weight, and the partnership at last had a better balance.

After I had been in the practice for a couple of years I was asked by Bristol University to take medical students for two weeks at a time so as to give them a taste of general practice. They would live with us and during the fortnight would be shared out amongst the other partners to get a taste of our differing styles of practice. It slowed down the surgeries a treat, but was fun and being asked why one had come to that conclusion or made that decision was good for us and stimulating. The baton for taking this on was in time passed around the partners. We were offered an invitation to process in one's academic robes in Bristol, at a degree ceremony, as a reward. Not an invitation any of us had the time or the desire to accept.

The medical students that came to us were a varied bunch of people, most of them impressive and well orientated human beings who were interested in the patients as people, not just walking examples of interesting pathology and, not unreasonably, often somewhat diffident in their approach to the human beings that they were meeting for the first time. One young woman impressed me that she was made of the right stuff for learning to be a medical practitioner. We were visiting a recently widowed little woman who was not feeling well. We were sitting on each side of her bed and she was describing her symptoms to me when she suddenly burst into tears and said, "Oh, I do miss Ivor so." As I put my arm around her shoulder, I was delighted to feel the medical student's arm come round from the other side. She had the right attitude to her future career.

I once had an American medical student with me for the day. During one of the surgeries that he was with me, a young man, who I had delivered eighteen years before and looked after all his life, came in with a very badly bruised forefinger. He was able, with considerable pain, to flex it nearly fully, so with the patient present I pontificated to the visitor that having that degree of movement made it very unlikely that it was fractured. In the USA, I continued pompously, you lot would X-ray it to protect yourself from being sued as a defensive measure. Why, I continued, shoot X-rays into his bone marrow to protect yourself, rather than for the benefit of the patient. The American was impressed and concurred. Two days later the lad came back in with his finger still a real mess and now totally immobile. Luckily for me the American student had left by then. I got it X-rayed, which showed a fracture. When I disclosed this to the patient he said, "I could sue you, doc." "But you are not going to, are you?" I said hopefully. "Not this time," was his reply.

One of the younger partners became a "trainer" of future general practitioners so we started to get qualified doctors into the practice as "trainees" now, more appealingly, called "registrars". These doctors stayed with the practice for varying lengths of time, up to six months or so and when on call would lodge with the duty doctor and take responsibility for the evening and night's work. When they stayed with us I usually managed to take a few pence off them playing backgammon.

Standard days

My day always started at 8.00am with a visit to our cottage hospital. A short ward round and often a bit of minor surgery - "lumps and bumps" to excise before the main surgery started at 9.00am. At that hour the inpatients were all still in their night clothes and still in their beds, which made it much easier to examine them than when they were already up and probably fully dressed. It disconcerted the nursing staff at first, but they soon acknowledged the practicality of the change in routine.

One morning in my early days here, as I came into the hospital the Matron asked me in to see her in her office. She was a large and stately Irish woman with a lovely sense of compassion as well as a great sense of humour. She started without any preamble, "I know that when you come in your mind is full and you are thinking about your patients and how they are, but it would be nice if you could say good morning to the staff." A lesson was learnt.

At that time the town's vicar was paid to be the hospital chaplain and was extremely idle, hardly ever earning his retainer. Matron asked our senior partner, who had the hospital cheque book in his charge, what they should do (no layers of management in those days). He wrote a brief letter to the vicar - "Dear Vicar, I understand that you have resigned as hospital chaplain, I therefore do not enclose a cheque". Funnily enough, the very next day the vicar arrived!

She was a superb and a "hands-on" nurse in spite of her senior status. When she was away the place became edgy and sometimes the staff fell out with each other. On her return from an absence the staff would go frowning into her office one by one to have their say and would always came out with a smile. I would go in and say, "All back to normal, Mary?" "Yes," she would say, "but it was like Paddy's Market in here, the Flanagan chasing the Banshee." She was well deserving of the respect that the whole town had for her. Before she retired we arranged for her to be invited to a Buckingham Palace Garden Party to which Ann and I were also were invited. We all went up by train together, had a lovely day, which was a thrill for her and us. Later on as she said that the Garden Party was the high point of her very successful career. Everyone was delighted when she stayed on in the town after her retirement.

Once the morning surgery was finished there was usually time for a cup of coffee and with it a pack of repeat prescriptions to sign. Then there was the visiting list to take on. Lots of them probably unnecessary, by today's standards. There would be numerous new visits plus the follow-up ones and the chronic sick to see, often fifteen and more in the day. Few people had cars or telephones and public transport was poor so that many of the visits were needed for those reasons. Routine checks were needed, for instance if a patient was taking digitalis it was important to check frequently on their pulse rate so as to confirm that the dose that they were taking was adequate, or not too large, and did not need adjusting. The terminally ill and their families needed all the support that regular visits provided and the palliative care could be adjusted when needed without crises occurring.

We had zoned the practice into different areas and had routine days for visiting these, which the patients knew and respected for demands other than for emergency visits. These days were often allied to the day of a branch surgery, which in the early days usually took place in a volunteer's front room. This was always a female, who would be paid, by the practice, for the privilege. These noble women seemed to enjoy the occasions when the surgery took place. At one branch surgery when I went into the waiting room to collect the next patient, if the most amusing local character was in residence, there would be considerable reluctance to leave the room to see the doctor and miss the gossip. "I am sure that you were next, it is not my turn," would be the refrain.

Once I was asked to call in on a council house on a Tuesday, which was the day I did a branch surgery in the area. After finishing the surgery I arrived at the house where the patient's wife told me that her husband had been in distress since Sunday with chest pain which sounded cardiac in origin. I went upstairs to his bedroom and as I said hello to him he died. He was on a very soft springy bed which would have been impossible to do CPR on, so I unceremoniously dragged him to the floor and set about the CPR. Alas it was useless and the considerate man died, probably because he did not want to put the doctor out of his known routine, and waited too long for help. Most upsetting.

One afternoon I was in the middle of a busy branch surgery in my most remote village when a message came through that I was urgently needed in a house five miles away, where I had seen an old lady three days before. She had had a minor sore throat and I had reassured her that it would be normal again in three days, did not give her a prescription, and told her to let me know if it did not get better.

These two sisters had had interesting working lives and the eldest, also the obvious boss, had been the headmistress of a City of London girls' school. When she had retired she was made a Freeman of the City of London. She certainly stood on her dignity. On getting this call I raced around to the village in which they lived leaving the patients waiting in the surgery. I was worried about what diagnosis I might have missed on my earlier visit. On my arrival at their home I found her and her sister enjoying a cosy cup of tea with scones and a sponge cake. When I asked what the crisis was they replied that there was no crisis, but they thought that I was a very casual young man not to have come back to see that my patient was better and had decided to teach me a lesson. I pointed out that I had left ten people sitting in a waiting room because of their action and left. They changed doctors the next day.

A young man who had lodgings with an elderly widow had slipped a disc and was flat on his back, immobile and in agony. In his circumstances he needed to be admitted to the cottage hospital. The snag was that at the time the ambulance service was on strike and there was no possible way that he could sit in a car. I rang up the undertakers and asked if they could help by transporting him to the hospital for me. They were delighted to oblige and tactfully arrived with their van and a stretcher rather than using the hearse.

I was called out of a distant branch surgery some weeks later on a glorious spring day. At the far end of the practice, some ten miles away, a solidly reliable patient of mine had suddenly started to behave in a totally bizarre manner and had left her home and was last seen walking rapidly northwards. As I followed the given directions, the banks were filled with primroses and the countryside quite beautiful. I finally came upon her striding vigorously up the lane towards the main road. I drew alongside, stopped the car and said, "Olive, I heard that you were in a muddle so came to see how you were." I invited her to get in, to which she agreed without hesitation, and I drove back towards our cottage hospital, talking to her en route. It became obvious that she was having an acute psychotic breakdown and needed institutional care. As I slowed down to turn into the sharp narrow hospital entrance she opened the car door, whilst we were still in motion, and without saying a word, got out and raced off down the street. One of her sons lived in a small terraced house in the town and I was sure that she would make for his house. I rang the Duly Authorised Officer, who in those days had the responsibility, alongside a doctor and the family, of committing mentally ill people to hospital against their will. My bloke was on holiday but an obliging stand-in said that he would help and we arranged to meet at her son's address. When we got there, sure enough, there was my patient enjoying a cup of tea. Her son was giving off all sorts of distress signals at his normally rational mother's bizarre behaviour. We explained to her that she was ill and needed to be admitted to hospital and it would be better for her to go voluntarily rather than being forced to be admitted. She readily agreed to this as long as she could take a large bottle of orange squash with her. There was an instant bustling about and a glass bottle full of orange squash was produced and, clutching this, she got into the back seat of the DAO's car and to our mutual relief was driven away to the mental hospital. I went back to finish my surgery.

During that evening surgery I took a call from the DAO, not a happy man. When they were halfway to the hospital she had hit him over his bald head with the glass bottle of orange squash and left the car. She then waved down a passing car that happened to contain four Royal Marines, saying that she was being kidnapped. Now Royal Marines are trained for instant unhesitating action. As the DAO got out of his car, blood streaming from his scalp wound, they flattened him, spread him out and pinned him down. It took some time to convince them that he was on an errand of mercy, but eventually Olive's psychotic behaviour persuaded them that she did need the hospital care that he had been trying to get them to believe that she needed. Soon he and Olive were sharing an ambulance, she to a psychiatric bed and he to a casualty department. His closing words to me were, "That is the last time I ever do you a favour."

By 1975 there were still a few houses in my practice that did not have an electricity supply; one of them was in a terraced street of cottages in the town, and another an isolated brick and thatched farm house, not the usual cob walls that most Devon thatched houses had. When it was built it must have been important, for the stairs, thankfully, had wide and shallow treads.

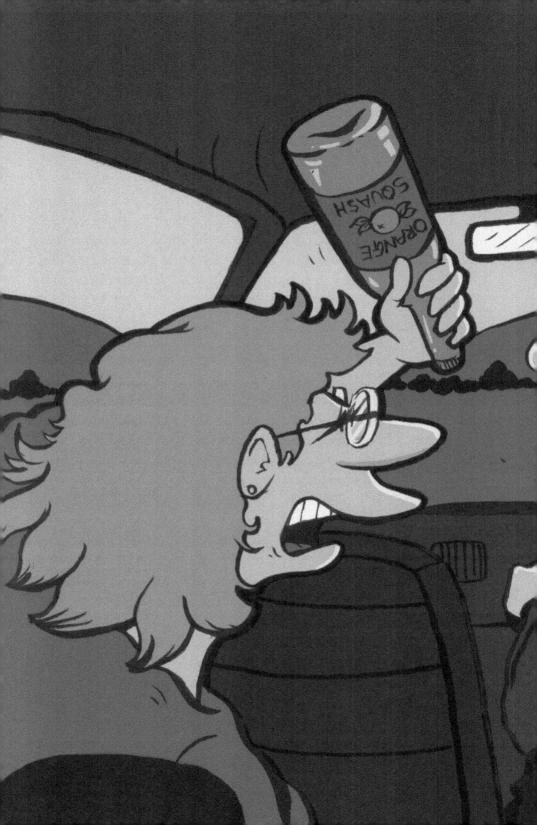

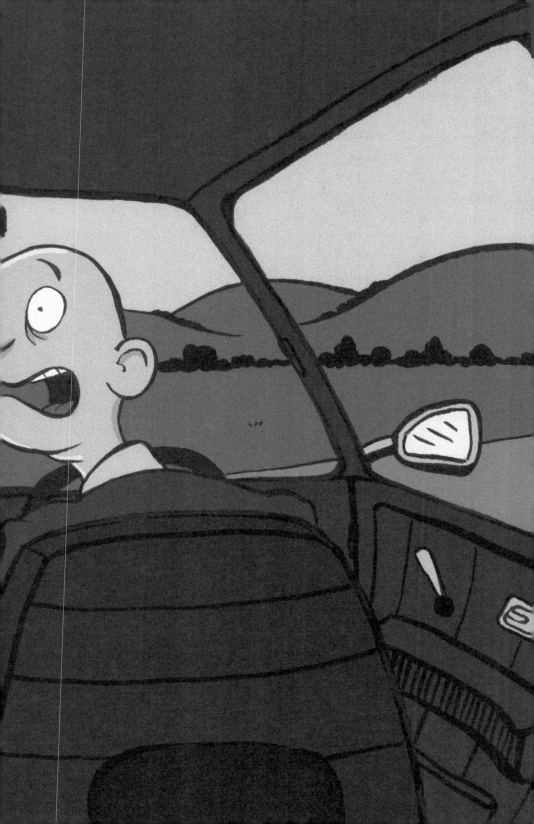

The town house inhabitants, both elderly, did not like the idea that there might be a leak of electricity from the light so had refused to have the supply connected. The sight of a steep wooden staircase being climbed by an eighty-plus-year-old-person carrying a paraffin lamp in a shaky hand was terrifying.

The inhabitants of the thatched farmhouse, two brothers and two sisters, all in their eighties, had refused the offer of an electricity supply on the grounds of cost. They still drew their water from a sacking-clad pump in the cobbled yard and cooked over the wood fire in the inglenook, the cooking pots hanging from hooks into the smoke. The fireplace was surrounded by two straight-backed wooden settles and the floor was of bare flagstones with a jute sack acting as a hearthrug. Their dwelling and lifestyle seemed unchanged from that of the seventeenth century or even earlier. Their cardiac health was a bit shaky and I visited every month to keep an eye on them and to monitor the effects of their digitalis dosage. In a room next to the kitchen were butter churns and cheese presses now no longer in use as the only livestock that they now owned was one cow.

I was called there one night because the elder brother was having breathing difficulties which turned out to be due to left-sided heart failure. I ascended the stairs behind one of his sisters who carried the candle in a trembling hand. Finding him in the semi-darkness deep in a Devon featherbed was difficult, but anyway the problem was soluble and he survived for another year or two.

Two days later I was giving a lecture on computer records to some London GPs and was going to stay the night with a colleague of my student days who was now a consultant surgeon at St Thomas' Hospital. When I arrived at the porters lodge to meet him he had left a message that he was held up and suggested that while waiting for him I visit the then fashionably new Intensive Care Unit, where an old friend of mine was the Sister in charge. She was showing me round when we came upon a bed on which lay an unconscious woman, with ten tubes and wires coming in or going out of her and various oscilloscopes were tracing out data. She was surrounded by nine white-coated doctors grouped silently around the bed. Oh Brave New World. The man nearest me was labelled Consultant Anaesthetist. I asked him what his role was. He replied succinctly, "Referee." A somewhat different style of medicine, compared with that practiced by me two nights before.

Before we had our in car wirelesses I arrived at a branch surgery at 11.00am one morning to find the local postmistress at the door with a message from our local obstetric unit saying that a girl in labour with her first baby was failing to make progress. I told the few people in the waiting room that I would probably be some time, but that I would call back as soon as could, and then left for the hospital. When I got there the babe's head was transverse across the woman's pelvis and would only be able to advance if the head was rotated through ninety degrees. I failed to rotate the head manually so needed to give the young woman a nerve block and turn the baby's head with Keilland's forceps. This was not without risk but all went well and a sweet little baby girl was delivered.

Nineteen years later when I was lecturing on general practice to nurses in training at the local district hospital, I was delighted to see the baby that I had delivered that distant morning grinning up at me from the front row. No brain damage there.

By the time the episiotomy was repaired and all sorted out at the obstetric unit and the baby girl comfortably in her mother's arms, it was after one o'clock before I returned to the branch surgery. There was no one left waiting to see me, but two messages had been left. The first message was a very cross one from a retired barrister saying that he knew that I was on the golf course in dereliction of my duty. The second message was a request to visit an old lady in an isolated cottage in a wood about two miles away. I immediately drove round to be welcomed by the old lady who smiled nicely and said how kind I was to call on her because she could not think of anyone else she could ask to post her letter. I was thoroughly relieved to find that there was no problem to solve and no thinking to be done, so took the letter and put it in the next post box that I came to.

There were always a few patients who needed the moral rather than the physical support of their doctor. Often a widow would latch on to her doctor as a solid reliable support, and show little kindnesses such as baking a cake for the doctor's children. One sweet woman, recently widowed, who needed to be appreciated, baked the most wonderful cakes which she would present to the surgery staff for their coffee breaks. She also made and gave her delicious cakes to the various charity jumble sales cake stalls, including the Cat's Protection Society.

A few days after one of these sales she came to see me in the surgery pale and trembling with fear, though she had calmly and efficiently looked after both her husband and her crabby mother-in-law when they were dying at her home. I had never seen her in such a state before. She tearfully told me that she might have to go to prison. She went on to say that a very young public health inspector had called on her that morning. Her landlord had just had a new bathroom fitted for her cottage and she imagined that the purpose of his visit was to inspect the new room and pass it as fit for the purpose. But not a bit of it. He said that he had been told by a person, who wished to remain anonymous, that she made cakes for sale and that she had a cat that came into her kitchen. He finished with the words, "Let me tell you that if one cat hair is ever found in one of your cakes, you, Madam, are for the high jump." She interpreted this as a gaol sentence. I was so angry about this bullying of a totally inoffensive woman that I rang our two local councillors and the council's Head of Public

Health and demanded that the young man should return and apologise. I am pleased to say that he was made to do just that. A nice thing coming out of this episode was that our staff all asked her to bake them cakes to buy as a gesture of solidarity.

As the years went by the increasing number of young single mothers who showed a lack of demonstrable affection and comfort for their children was most upsetting. I recall one evening visit to a house where a single mother lived with her two small daughters, then aged three and four. One of the girls was feverish, which was why I had been called to visit. I rang the doorbell and was let in by their mother who had a cigarette in her hand. She leant against the sitting room doorjamb, arms folded, and said, gesturing with her cigarette towards the two frightened little girls, clad only in their vests, huddled up against one another on the sofa, "She's in there." No sitting the child on her knee, not a word of explanation to them about me, not a hint of cuddling or comforting for either of them. The sad thing is that as they themselves were not being taught how to be affectionate they could well grow up unable to show affection and be able to cuddle their children when they themselves become mothers.

This may hurt a little...

Complaints and problems

Accusations against doctors are not always fair. Once when I was doing a surgery a colleague poked his head round my door and asked if I could spare a moment to help. A patient was complaining that this particular doctor had given her son an overdose of medicine. I went with him into his consulting room where a furious-looking mother was sitting with her small son on her knee. I asked her what the problem was. She said that the day before she had brought her son, who had earache, to see the doctor. After examining the child he had prescribed a penicillin medicine, to take a teaspoonful four times a day. "It was too big a dose," she said, grabbing her child's ear and pulling his head sideways. "Look - it overflowed when I poured a teaspoonful into his ear." Sure enough, the red stain of the penicillin medicine showed that it had overflowed!

During one surgery the husband of a patient that I had seen the previous day made an appointment to see me and arrived in a state of fury. He opened the consultation with the aggressive statement, "How dare you prescribe whitewash for my wife." I was puzzled because all I had prescribed was a white powder (magnesium trisilicate) for his wife's indigestion. Why did he think that she had been given whitewash? It transpired that the pharmacist had said to her, as he handed over the packet, "Are you going to whitewash the scullery with this?" I had to explain that this local pharmacist had a great sense of fun and all he was doing was teasing her. The husband left somewhat mollified, whilst I immediately rang the chemist to ask him to be more careful of whose leg he was pulling. Teasing him, I said that I was prescribing a complicated ointment for him to prepare which was difficult to make and would make the whole pharmacy stink for days.

I had seen a late middle aged man a few times with vague chest pains, the pain was not anginal in character and an ECG had shown no abnormality. A month or so later he dropped dead whilst shopping. His widow was a frequent habitué of one of the local pubs and it was reported back to me that she was often heard in the pub saying that I had killed her husband. I was at the time looking after the husband of another female regular of the same pub, who was dying of a recurrent stomach cancer. After he had died his wife told me that she would put up a notice in the pub saying, "Dr Jeremy did not kill my husband".

I have never been a believer in ghosts or telepathy but have two incidents in my mind of when I suddenly felt that my presence was urgently required. The first occasion was when a patient, who had already borne three children without any problem, was in labour at home. During my morning visiting rounds some three miles away I suddenly felt that I needed to check up on how the labour was going. I drove back to the town and let myself into the house to meet a white-faced father hurtling down the stairs. "Thank God you are here," he exclaimed, "I was just on my way to the telephone box to call you. The midwife wants you urgently." I rushed up the stairs to find the boy baby delivered but with white asphyxia. I had some difficulty getting him breathing but in the end all was well and he grew up to be a really good solid citizen. I am also certain that if my arrival and been only slightly later he might not have survived.

The second occasion was when I was on holiday and was returning with Ann from a shopping trip. We were close to the house of an elderly patient, who was also a friend, and had not been well when I started my holiday. The thought came to me that I must call in and see how he was. I was surprised when the front door was opened by his married daughter who lived many miles away. When she saw me, she said, "The surgery said that you were on holiday." They had called for a visit as his health had deteriorated.

He was dying and his living-in helper was also very ill. She had pneumonia and needed hospitalisation, which I fixed up. The ambulance arrived to pick her up and take her to hospital, and she was loaded into it and driven off. As we heard the noise of the ambulance crossing the cattle-grid, my patient died.

A medical student once told me that I was like a chameleon changing my persona with each different patient, sometimes jokey, sometimes grave and all nuances in between those extremes. I think that, subconsciously, I was suiting my attitude to what I felt that the patient needed. Of course if you got it wrong you did not make a friend. I once saw the patient of a holidaying partner with a minor problem and, summing him up wrongly, went into great detail with what I thought was happening. His response was not flattering. "I hate seeing you; you get me in such a muddle. My doctor just says, "Nothing much wrong with you, come back if it does not get better."

The so-called "heart sink" patients present a challenge. A few of one's patients never seemed to respond favourably to whatever one tried to do for them, and returned again and again to challenge one's ingenuity and patience. I found that the frustration that they caused was mitigated if at each consultation one scored them from 1 to 10 in aggravation. When one called them in, one could say to oneself, "At the last consultation they were level 6, I bet that they cannot beat that today". However I always tried to take their complaints seriously. Usually, though, their problems were only due to extreme anxiety, but anyway the biggest hypochondriac can still get appendicitis. One patient was so persistent in always saying that I never got anything right etc. etc. that I eventually told him that if I was so useless he might be better off with another doctor. "But you're my doctor," he said with determination, and from then on I seemed to get everything right as far as he was concerned.

A young man who had lived in the town for a couple of years was in that age group that hardly ever needed medical attention unless they have had an accident. He has been married for about a year when he came to see me complaining of a sore throat. Yes, he had a red throat, but must have had just the same on several occasions without feeling the need to see a doctor. There must be a hidden agenda, but asking various chatty questions about his new wife's cooking and married life drew no response, and he left with me feeling that there was unfinished business that I had not drawn out of him.

A week later he came back, this time accompanied by his wife. He started the conversation with the dread remark, which usually precedes a story of tragedy, "You are going to laugh at this" and then explained that they had never been able to have intercourse. I examined her and found that she had a very tough hymen which I manually stretched in his presence and showed him what to do. I delivered the baby a year later. Imagine the courage that it took to tell another male about that problem. No wonder he came in to first suss me out and imagine how differently things could have turned out if I had been dismissive about his sore throat.

I had one man who fitted into the heart sink category; every cold could be pneumonia or tuberculosis, every headache a brain tumour or meningitis. One day he came in with a significant painless obstructive jaundice. The diagnosis showed that it was due to a rare tumour in his common bile duct which was blocking the flow of bile into his small bowel and hence the jaundice. The surgeons were unable to remove the cancer, but made a permanent drain from his gall bladder through to the skin. He came out with a small bag stuck to his abdominal wall to catch the flow of bile, and his jaundice receded. His three sons came to see me and, not unreasonably, said that knowing dad as they did, I was not to tell him what was wrong. My reply was that he was bound to ask and I would not lie to him... if he did. Sure enough, his first question was to ask why he was left like that. I told him that the cancer could not be cut out, but what had made him ill was the build-up of bile in his body, which was a problem now solved. I used the analogy of a watch that could be dirty but still ticking if nothing vital was involved. He seemed satisfied and from then on was calm and brave. He lived, staying well, for another two years. When he died the sons told me that he and mum had had the best years of their marriage as he had stopped fussing. The worst had happened and there had been no need to be anxious any more.

I had been called to a retired farmer and his wife one day and had what seemed a routine consultation with them, so was surprised when the following day, my senior partner said that they had rung him to say that they never wanted to have me in their house again. He had had no explanation from them, and I could not work out what I had done to cause this reaction. A year later when I was on call for the weekend I got a message asking for a doctor to call on them. Rather nervously I attended, dealt with the matter without any fuss of any kind, and set out to leave the house. "Which doctor are you?" I was asked, "I am Dr Jeremy," I answered. "No you are not," was the immediate reply!

In the 1950s and 1960s there was an over-respectful attitude towards the medical profession, and the reasons for actions taken by doctors were rarely questioned. When I was doing my first house surgeon job my consultant performed a major operation on a man with a large cancer in his rectum. The operation involved excising his rectum completely leaving him with a permanent colostomy. On the ward round a day or two later, my boss came to his bedside and told him that all he had had was a tiny little ulcer and nothing to worry about. "Thank you, sir," was the grateful reply.

This attitude persisted for some time, the doctors shying away from breaking bad news and the patient often being too respectful to ask important questions. The scales fell from my eyes early on in my general practice career when I was called on a Saturday evening to see a farmer's wife in pain. When I went into the farmhouse the stressed family was assembled around the kitchen table and in hushed tones told me that she had "Cancer" and did not know it. I went up the stairs to where the sick woman was in bed. On examining her I noted the scar from a breast amputation. She was suffering from bad pain in her spine, due to the spread of the cancer. Previous explanations had been evasive and full of half-truths and she did not know what to think or believe.

I went down to the car to collect some diamorphine, telling the family that I was going to discuss her future truthfully with her. Back in her room I told her the truth of what was happening to her. I reassured her that the pain could be controlled. I then gave her the injection of diamorphine, and said that I would be back in the morning to check up on her. Uncertainty is much more damaging than knowledge. On returning the next morning the whole atmosphere in the house was different, she had had a good night's sleep, but best of all she knew what she had to face and was relieved to know the truth, and her children were happy that the time for evasion and half-truths was gone and their relationship could be honest.

The flip side of this type of over-adulation of the doctor was that one's behaviour was constantly monitored and talked about; you were a big fish in a small puddle. A year after the old patrician doctor had retired he rang the surgery to say that he would be in the town on a fleeting visit and hoped to see the three of us before lunch in a local pub. We duly arrived; two of us had a soft drink and the other had a half pint of beer. Timing was difficult as my wife was in labour with our fourth child in the nearby large hospital. I got in to see her just after the baby was born and then dashed back to start the five o'clock surgery. The first patient in, an elderly spinster, started the consultation with the words, "I am surprised to see you here, Doctor." I thought that the jungle drums were pretty efficient and that she was referring to the new birth, but she followed up with the words, "I hear that you were drinking in a pub at lunch time."

After that I never went into a local pub unless called to an emergency, such as one when a spectator at a darts match dropped dead. I arrived to find the body lying prone near the "oche" with the darts teams and about fifteen spectators standing around looking down at the still figure. I started resuscitation, with this audience watching intently, until the ambulance arrived, when I gave it over to the ambulance men, no paramedics in those days, so that I could look at his optic fundi with an ophthalmoscope. I could see the retinal arteries "cattle-trucked" which meant that death had already occurred; continuing the resuscitation was pointless, so we stopped it. A discussion then took place amongst the teams and spectators, the nub of it being how the dead fan would not have wanted the match stopped as he was such a supporter of the team, who anyway were leading in the league match. The match, needless to say, continued after the ambulance, the body and I had gone. I never found out the result.

If I ever feel that I have been unlucky or that something in life has been unfair, I think of a fine intelligent female patient who I looked after for years, and what a wretched hand life dealt her. She had been a petty officer in the WRENS and was married in her thirties to an ex-Royal Navy deep sea clearance diver who was now working for the oil industry in the Persian Gulf. After a year or so of marriage, their baby girl was born. A little before Christmas he returned to his diving job in the Gulf. The day after Boxing Day she called me saying that their daughter was ill and could I visit. The child was very ill with pneumonia, and the mother had not called over Christmas, not wanting to be a nuisance. The little girl reached hospital alive, but sadly died at seven o'clock that evening.

The next disaster for her occurred the summer following while her husband was back home on holiday. The couple, with two friends, hired a small boat and went fishing off the coast. After a while, having caught nothing, he said that he would put on his scuba kit and have a look at what was going on "down there". He slipped into the water with his marker buoy and shortly after the buoy bobbed free, which did not cause a worry, but by the time that his air would be running low they started to get alarmed. The engine was started, they buoyed the spot that they were at and then circled around in increasing circles, while alerting the Coastguards, all to no avail.

No trace of his body was ever found in spite of an intensive and thorough search being made. After hearing what had happened I called on her, to see if there was anything I could do to help. She asked me if I could ask the driver of a car parked outside her house in the small housing estate to move as he was upsetting her. I asked her who he was and she said that he was from the local press and wanted a story. When she had told him that she had nothing to say he told her that he would stay there until she did have something to say. I went out and told him that she was upset by his presence and was not prepared to have an interview now or later. He said that if she did not give him a story he would get the national press involved and then she would learn what harassment was. I then lost my temper and told him what I thought of him, to which he replied that he knew who I was and from now on any story about me, and also the school of which I was Chairman of Governors, he would portray in a negative light. He then settled down to stay. I telephoned a lawyer friend who said that getting an injunction would draw attention and only worsen the situation. I was advised to ring the editor and complain to him. I duly telephoned and spoke to the wife of the editor, telling her what I thought of the man's behaviour, little realising that the hyena in the car was in fact the editor. She did eventually get hold of him and called him off, and I duly got hostile headlines from him for ages afterwards.

This poor woman was left feeling guilty about the delay in calling me when her daughter was ill as well, and now she had the ghastliness of there never being a proper closure in the matter of her husband's disappearance and later his legally accepted death. The final awful piece in the accumulating tragedy of her life was that she developed Huntington's chorea to add misery to the last years of her life, before her descent into madness and an early and merciful death.

I was looking after Archie, a retired bricklayer, who was reaching the end of his life suffering from a spread of a stomach cancer. I visited twice weekly keeping a close eye on his pain relief and other medication. Hanging in their living room was a striking drawing of an attractive demure young woman, beautifully drawn and with the signature R.Whistler scrawled on it. It was a drawing of his wife, Edie, done many years before, when she was working as a young housemaid at a large house nearby. The young artist had asked her to sit for the drawing. I mischievously suggested to Archie that there could have something between them to have created such a beautiful drawing. "She was never as good as she pretended," was his answer, to which her reply was a smiling, "You men!" This exchange between the three of us was developed over the further few weeks that he lived. After he had died I saw no more of her as, though I was Archie's doctor, his wife was the patient of our senior partner. One evening, several years later, there was a knock on the door and standing there with a brown paper parcel was Edie's brother. "Edie died last week," he said, "and before she died she said that I was to give you this." 'This' was the Whistler drawing of Edie. He then said, "She so enjoyed Archie and you teasing her about it that she wanted you to have it after she died. So here it is." It was very gratefully received and hangs in pride of place in our house.

Outside interests

I was a poor but enthusiastic cricketer and immediately joined the town cricket club. It was difficult to play in many away matches because of my then on-call commitments but I could manage the home games. I was not the only player liable to be called away as our most reliable bowler was a retained fireman. He would park his bicycle by the gate to the cricket field and if the fire siren went so did he, throwing the ball down in mid-over and cycling at top speed to the fire station, with the time of his return totally uncertain. There were the, not unusual, internecine wars and rivalries going on at the club and the following year I was made captain, as being a newcomer I was more likely to be seen as a neutral figure in the sniping contests, rather than because I was a good cricketer.

One of the team once arrived at a partner's surgery with a black eye. He told the doctor that he had been playing cricket and been hit by a bat. "You must have been fielding very close in," said the partner. "No, I was in the outfield," came the reply, "and it was one of those little furry flying things that got me in the eye."

Two years later I was able to hand over to a much more competent skipper, and continued to play, and many years later ended up as the club chairman. An old lady in the town very kindly volunteered to knit me a pair of cricket socks. Her son, a keen cricketer himself, tried to persuade her to put a row of ducks around the top of them, which she loyally refused to do.

The absurd over-respect for the figure of the doctor was manifest in that our then cricket club chairman would not let my wife and I run the second hand clothes stall at the club's winter Saturday jumble sale, but we were allowed to man the cake stall. He also would not let me help at the weekly fundraising tombola as he deemed it not a suitable activity for a doctor to be seen doing.

We local doctors were also asked to judge fancy dress competitions, light celebratory bonfires and other quasi-ceremonial duties. Thank goodness there were no beautiful baby competitions to judge, when one's life would have been at risk of death by a lynch mob comprised of the mothers of the losers. All these activities helped us to be more use in our role as local doctors. One would hear that a man was losing his job; that a businessman was looking for a new secretary, that a certain house was up for sale, or the gossip that a marriage was a bit rocky. Lots of background information would come our way, much of it docketed away to be useful in suggesting to an employer that a good bloke was looking for a job or why a usually cheerful character was looking so miserable.

Both of our sons belonged to the junior sections of local rugby and cricket clubs, whilst our two daughters excelled at the hockey and tennis clubs. I ran the junior section of the cricket club for a short time before a better cricketer and coach took over. Later a patient with myasthenia gravis, a muscle weakening disease, told me how bored she got being so immobile. I introduced her to Test Match Special on the radio. I made her a chart of the fielding positions and a glossary of cricket terms and she became a great enthusiast. As a reward she joined me up as a member of Somerset County Cricket Club at their ground in Taunton. Once on holiday, I was watching a county game when, Ian Botham, whilst fielding at slip, was hit in the part that really hurts by a ball that bounced awkwardly in front of him. He started to laugh, then went a deathly pale, fell down, and had to be helped from the field. There came a call on the loudspeaker. "Is there a doctor in the pavilion?" Seeing no one else move, I answered the call and was ushered into the home side's dressing room. I am glad to report that there was no serious damage was found.

The family and I spent many happy hours at the Somerset ground. One time my wife Ann was having difficulty in manoeuvring her long estate car out of their small congested car park. My offer to help was being curtly refused when the giant West Indian fast bowler, Joel Garner, appeared, still in his whites. "Hold it, Mam," he said, and with that he put his back against the car, grabbed the rear wheel arch and lifted the back of the car up and moved it a foot clear. Here was an international sportsman risking injury to help a damsel in distress, what a lovely man.

I also played squash which had the huge advantage that one could get plenty enough exercise in forty minutes so it did not intrude on family time. I played until I was fifty years old when during a close-fought game my heart had a short spell of irregular beats which stopped the game and all future games. I did continue to play in the occasional game of cricket when the team was short or playing for parents against the school and other relaxed games. I only once played in the same team as both my sons and rather disgraced myself. My elder son was bowling fast medium pace and put me in a fielding position which I, in my wisdom, thought was in no-man's-land, so I moved myself deeper and needless to say the catch came to where I should have been and I never got to it. I was not a very popular father at that time.

Our small town was an urban district council until, in 1972, a local government reorganisation joined us into a large conglomeration. In 1969 I became a candidate for election to be a local councillor and was elected. I ended up as chairman of the Public Health and Housing Committee, where I was able to achieve a number of the changes that I had wanted to see, mainly the modernisation of some of the older council houses which, even in 1969, had no hot water systems, only a copper by the back door under which a fire had to be lit in order to heat the water. Each house had only one two pin electric socket on the landing to deal with the whole upstairs and none of them had a proper larder. The cost to the ratepayers was nothing at all, as there were government grants available for those specific purposes. At another time I was laughed at by the other councillors for suggesting that car parking spaces ought to be made for the council houses. Council house tenants will never own cars, I was told. Now there are often two or three cars per household.

The over-respectful approach to doctors was sometimes the cause of amusement. When there was to be a rise in the rents paid by the council house tenants, I arranged two meetings to explain what was happening. There was to be an afternoon meeting for the elderly and an evening meeting for the working men. The afternoon meeting went off well but the evening meeting was more challenging. After I had explained what was proposed one of my more bellicose patients rose from his seat and told me in no uncertain terms what he thought of my proposals. Immediately a furious little elderly woman, who had missed the afternoon meeting, leapt to her feet from the front row and rounded on him with the words, "Don't you dare speak to the doctor like that." The whole hall burst into laughter at her fury, changing the atmosphere wonderfully.

When the reorganisation of local government came I had no interest in giving up my evenings off to help administer the amalgamation of other small local towns, so did not stand for re-election. However while I was a councillor I had been nominated to be a school governor for the local Grammar School (where our four children received a first rate education) and also a trustee to two small local charities. I continued in these roles after ceasing to be on the council. After several years as a school governor I was elected as Chairman of Governors of the new Comprehensive School when it was formed from the existing excellent Grammar School. I continued in that role for several years. Not all of them easy and with school governors taking on more responsibilities there was a huge increase in paperwork. A wad of directives from the Ministry of Education arrived each week and the gold-plated interpretation of the same missives arrived a few days later from Devon County Council Education department. All had to be studied.

A small group of us parents with tiny children started the first playgroup at the town which saw me as the chairman during the time that our youngest daughter attended. When she left to go to primary school I resigned the post and our newest partner, who still had very small children, took on the job. All of us doctors took part in helping run various societies, trusts and clubs as part of our roles as local doctors. We were very much part of the local scene, big fish in a tiny puddle, which also gave us a good insight into the lives of our patients. I firmly believe that living in the community that we worked in was a necessary part of doing the job to the best of one's ability.

Our fortnight's holiday was always spent by the Helford River where my wife's generous uncle lent us his cottage and the use of his small boats. A friend of ours, while staying there with us, taught me to sail in their small dinghy, infecting me with the sailing bug. I had recently been left £100 by a patient whose wife I had looked after when she was dying of multiple myelomatosis, some two years before he died, so I bought a kit and over winter, helped by the family, built a Mirror dinghy. We had completed this project by early spring and were eagerly awaiting a chance to try her out.

I had a week's holiday planned in early April and was desperate to sail her, so my elder son, Charles, then eleven years old, and I trailed her to Lyme Regis and, ill-advisedly, launched her from the Cobb, into a brisk offshore wind. We had no sooner got out of the harbour than we capsized. We soon righted her and got back into her, by which time we were some way out to sea. We had a hard beat back to the harbour, which was difficult, but managed to capsize again, just in the mouth of the harbour. My son ended up about five yards from the steps on the end of the harbour wall, so naturally swam to them, leaving me holding onto the dinghy which I righted and then was blown out to sea again. Hampered by my life jacket, I could not board it by myself. Charles volunteered to jump in to help, but I shouted to him to run to the inshore lifeboat station and get help. After having spent the winter building her I was not going to abandon her so clung on. To slow down my rapid progress out to sea I turned her upside down again, but found that as I got colder it was harder to hold onto the hull, so had to turn her the right way up again, so that I could hold on by lodging my elbows over the transom, but with the sails still up this accelerated my departure out to sea. It was a huge relief to hear the maroons fired and to know that help was on the way.

I was heaved out of the water by the inshore lifeboat's competent crew after some twenty minutes in the water and they towed the Mirror back to the harbour. The sea had been extremely cold and I was shaking like a leaf with the cold. Charles and I were taken up to the local hospital to be warmed up and examined by the local lifeboat doctor. After warming baths we were both passed as fit and luckily all ended well, no thanks to my stupidity. However the local radio station gave graphic details of my rescue and to my extreme embarrassment the surgery phone lines were kept busy by people ringing up to find out if I was all right. To add to my shame a local newspaper produced an article headlined, "Eleven year old son swims two miles through heavy seas to rescue father". This resulted in several people saying that they had not realised that I could not swim! The RNLI got a heartfelt and well-earned donation.

After a few years of dinghy sailing my wife and I were invited to cruise to the Channel Islands and the Brittany coast in a friend's large sailing yacht and later I was asked to help crew the vessel in several offshore and cross channel races. Thus I gained enough experience to make two cruises as a watch officer with the Sail Training Association in their topsail schooner *Sir Winston Churchill*. On my second cruise we experienced hurricane (force 12) winds off Ushant, and were reported as missing in the *Daily Telegraph*. I had always wanted to see heavy weather and now, having seen it, do not want to meet it again. The shrieking noise of the wind in the rigging for hour after hour was all prevailing and exhausting, the sea was white with foam and the balls of spindrift, the size of small footballs, were flying by. Most of our sails were shredded and the life rafts were washed off into the sea. The weight of water coming aboard was enough to bend the steel rod, from which the anchor bell hung, six inches out of true. Two fully grown men could not pull it straight again. The force of the water also moved the companionway to the half deck out of position. This weather continued for some eight hours as we struggled to make our way west with the lee shore of Ushant getting closer on our starboard side until we were able to turn round the western corner of Ushant, and could then free off in the lee of Brittany, to race up the coast and anchor later in the shelter of Guernsey.

I sailed on her as a watch officer and the skipper preferred that I was not to be known as being a doctor, which suited me fine. However one of the boys in the crew had a fragment of grit blown into his right eye during the storm. This minute bit of grit had become stuck to his cornea and was extremely painful. There were no local anaesthetic eyedrops on board so there was no way the fragment could be lifted off his cornea on the ship. As we were anchored off Guernsey at the time, the skipper asked me to take him up to the hospital at St Peter Port so that they could deal with the matter. We got to the hospital and a charming newly qualified young female doctor was in charge of the Casualty Department. I explained to her that I was a doctor and had not been able to lift the grit off his cornea on the ship because of the lack of local anaesthetic eyedrops. She said that she had never seen the job done, and could I show her how to do it. I naturally said yes. The look on the poor boy's face when he saw his watch officer advancing on him with a sharp implement, while the white-coated doctor stood by to watch, was a picture.

Our small boat cruising had been such fun that we resolved to buy a small yacht. The friend who had infected me with the sailing bug came in with us, sharing the costs. We bought together a tough little 27 foot yacht which answered our needs well, and could sleep six at a squeeze. In those days we had no VHF radio, no life raft, no navigational electronics, just a trailing log, depth gauge, and compass. We navigated by dead reckoning when crossing the Channel, working out the tidal streams and speeds. How things have changed in the following years; when we finally sold our last yacht we had a heater, digital VHF, radar, a life raft and a chart plotter with a system called AIS which identified other shipping and almost told you the colour of their skipper's eyes.

Our first holiday with our little yacht saw us cross the Channel on a club race to Brittany, after which we cruised along the lovely Brittany coast. I later qualified as an Offshore Skipper and bit by bit the new clever navigation aids were added. After that we nearly always felt that we knew, and usually did know, exactly where we were, so the sense of triumph previously felt when one had made a good landfall went missing, but the reassurance of knowing where one was, especially in the event of poor visibility, made up for it. After seven years the growing children issued an ultimatum. "We can't stand up, our bunks are too small, and we have to breathe in and out in time. If you don't buy a larger yacht we will not sail with you", a splendid excuse to buy a bigger faster boat. This we did, buying a 32 foot Swedish yacht which sailed well and was infinitely more comfortable.

We were also involved in club racing with a crew making six of us, on our weekends off call, which was fun, and our holiday cruising range extended into the Bay of Biscay and across to the north Spanish coast. Often we had to set sail for home with a poor weather forecast because of the necessity to get back from holiday in time, as a partner would be champing on the bit, waiting for his turn to get away on holiday, as soon as we got back. This increased our experience and competence and confidence enough for Ann and I to plan for the two of us to cross the Atlantic in the year that I retired. This we successfully achieved.

Seven years later, with all the children away from home, we bought a heavy 36 foot ocean cruising yacht to make possible the intention of the ocean sailing we had planned for when I retired, and our racing days ended. I was fifty five years old at the time and had five years to go before my retirement at sixty. I was tired out, so we took a three month sabbatical, added a month of holiday to it and hired a locum to take my place in the practice. I resigned at that time from chairmanship of the school governors, leaving the school with an excellent new headmaster in charge. We spent the four months cruising around the British Isles in a leisurely manner learning our new vessel's ways. We had our family aboard for spells, which including meeting up with our first grandchild. Friends also joined us at intervals. We spent the longest time around the Western Highlands which that summer was blessed with wonderful weather. I came back to the practice thoroughly refreshed and once again full of ideas about the future and with a renewed appetite for work.

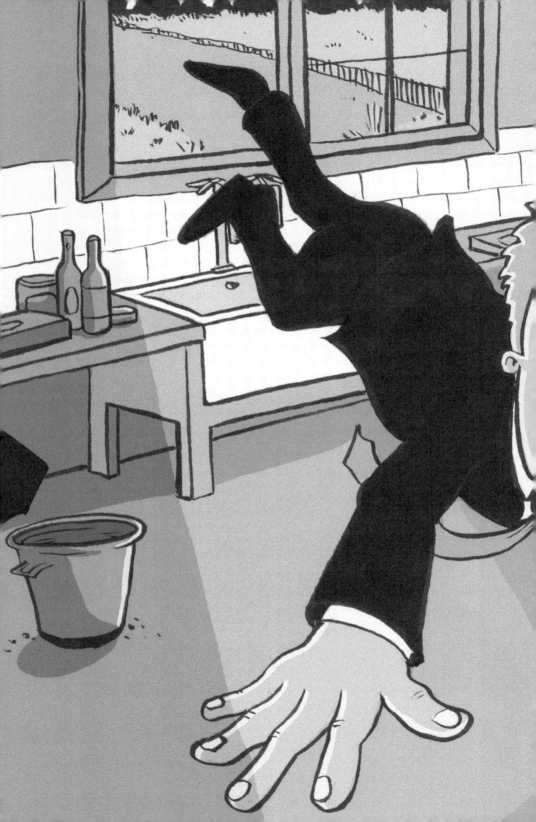

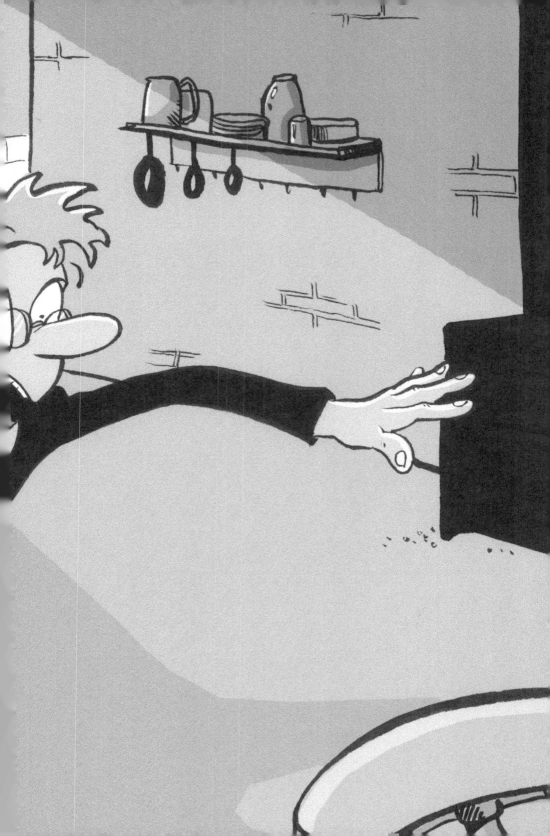

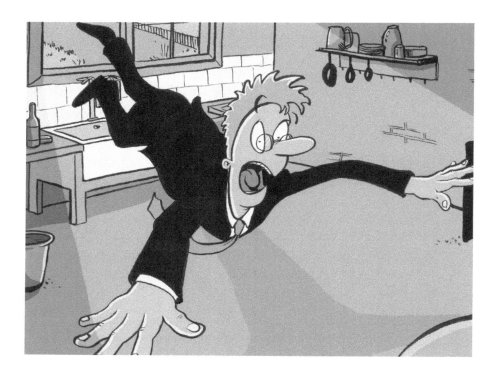

Breaking and entering

Not infrequently a neighbour would ring to say that their next-door neighbour had not appeared that day or that the milk had not been taken in off the doorstep, and could the doctor call and investigate. The first time this occurred was when I was delivering my elder two children to the door of the house where a splendid old teacher ran a pre-school class. On our arrival a small group of parents were waiting outside and told us that she was not answering the door. Old Bert who lived alongside appeared and said that she had been knocking all night, and he had thought that she must have been making something.

The scullery window was ajar so I said that I would break in through it. Old Bert pointed out that she usually bolted the door through into the rest of the house on the inside. Regarding him as an unreliable witness, I ignored him and got up and through the window which was over the sink. Stepping down from the window, I caught the turn-up of my trousers on one of the taps and measured my length on the floor. Needless to say the door was bolted, just as Bert had said that it would be. We called the police who broke down the front door to find the old lady on her bedroom floor having suffered a major stroke. The little school never reopened.

Once a call came in from a good neighbour; she was worried about a very deaf old lady, who had not taken in her milk or newspapers at the time that she usually did. Dutifully she had tried telephoning her with no success and was, not unreasonably, worried about her health. The policeman arrived and after trying the bell and hammering on the door, with great efficiency kicked in the door and he and I entered, fearing the worst. To our relief she was comfortably knitting by her fire, and seemed totally unfazed by the unannounced arrival of two large men.

She forgave us for damaging her front door and did not make a claim for the repair.

On another occasion I was called by the police to a house where a passer-by had seen through his widowed neighbour's large front window that he had not moved from his chair for twenty four hours. He had not responded to the window being tapped either. Indeed he had been dead for over twenty four hours. The smell of burning in the house was due to some charred and shrivelled sausages still cooking in the oven. The policeman suggested, with the mordant humour of those such as police and undertakers, who see death frequently, that the actual time of death might be calculated forensically by the size to which the sausages had shrunk.

The only time that I have ever seen a couple of undertakers thoroughly discomforted was when I was called urgently to a remote gypsy caravan. They had just put the body of a large man, who had died the night before, into his coffin and had then asked his widow if she would like to see him. She came into the room, looked at her husband's body, then she said, "Don't he look lovely?" at which point she dropped to the floor, dead herself. Familiar with death as they were, neither of them had ever seen anybody die and it had shaken both of them to the core.

On another occasion the postman, after getting home, rather late in the day, was worried that the newspaper was still in the door when he delivered the post to an elderly lady who lived in a cottage on the side of a hill, remote from any nearby dwelling. Eventually he decided that he had better do something about it so he telephoned the surgery to say perhaps somebody ought to check up that all was well. I was the nearest doctor to the house at that time, so was called up on the wireless to check up on her. I did not know her or her house, but found my way there after dark. I parked in the lane and walked up the narrow path to the front door. I banged on the door and stood back. A voice from above shouted, "Who's there?" I looked up and I saw, pointing at me out of an upstairs window, a large revolver held in a shaky elderly hand. I rapidly explained who I was and why I was there, to be told to go away as she was perfectly well. This instruction I rapidly obeyed.

The most bizarre event in my breaking and entering career occurred one January evening. Once again I was asked by the police to attend whilst they broke into a small terraced house in the town. This was lived in by a reclusive old lady, who kept herself to herself, and had not even registered as a patient with our practice. The neighbours did not know her name or anything about her. A concerned next-door neighbour had not seen or heard anything from her house for a few days so had called the police. The constable and I gathered in her tiny front garden and decided that the best route of entry would be through her front window. With minimum of damage we got in through the window into what appeared to be an empty room with no signs of life, though the fireplace had a burnt out fire in the grate. There were no pictures on the walls and just a battered armchair beside the fire and nothing decorative or comfortable in view. We moved through into the sparse empty kitchen, with just an old fashioned gas cooker, a clean empty sink and a bare, clean, scrubbed wooden table. Then we climbed on up the stairs to enter a bleak empty bedroom. This was again bare of any ornament or furniture other than a carefully well-made bed, and again no other sign of life.

The next room was both a shock and a surprise; it was totally unfurnished with a bare well-scrubbed floor, except that it was filled with row upon row of neatly lined up, new, untarnished zinc buckets, each one full of faeces. These were in various different stages of decomposition from fresh, to those covered in mould. Moving on to the next room, we discovered it full of more buckets with more of the same contents, but still no sign of a human being.

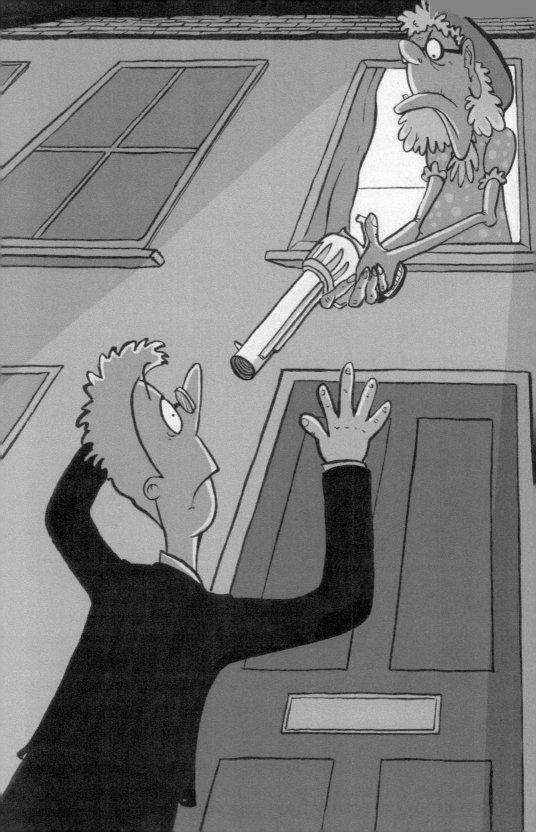

Obviously the lavatory had not worked and her solution to the problem had been to use a bucket and when it was full, put it aside, and buy another. This must have been going on for some time, judging by the number of buckets. As there were still no signs of the occupant in any part of the house, we returned to the front room and there we found, in a tiny space between the easy chair and the wall, a very small and a very dead body. It never ceases to amaze me how small a space a dead human being can occupy. Her death was from natural causes, but I never discovered who she was.

On another occasion the occupant of a council old people's bungalow had not been seen for several days. She was a staunch old lady who, before she retired, had been a cleaner at the local hospital for many years, so I knew her quite well. It had been known by the neighbours that she had not been well for some time and she had not been outside for days. Worried by this, they had eventually talked to her through her front door but could not get in as, in spite of being unlocked, the door was jamming. I managed to force the door open, having to push her supine body aside to get in. She was in a dreadful state of filth and mess, very ill but conscious. There was no way that she could be left in that condition. When the ambulance arrived she refused to be moved, and the ambulance men were properly reluctant to do so without her permission, which she would not give. I stated that if there was any comeback about moving her I would take the responsibility, so they took her down to the cottage hospital where she had worked so usefully for so many years. I went down later that afternoon after she had been cleaned up to check on how she was. The Sister in charge invited me to look at the bathtub that she had been washed in. The bottom of the bath was alive with hundreds of maggots that had been washed off her ulcerated back. She must have been lying on the floor of her house for days. She died the next day.

Another unusual episode occurred during a cold spell one winter. A retired teacher, who had never been married, had moved into a small bungalow in a small village in the north of our practice. She had entered into all the village functions and was well liked and respected as someone independent who knew her own mind and coped well with life as she grew older. What none of us had recognised was that under the familiar acceptable social façade was an increasing dementia. This came to light when her home help, who cleaned for her twice a week, could not get in one morning. She saw that the bathroom light in the bungalow was on, so went round to the window tapped on it and asked if she was alright. "I am in the bath," was the reply. The cleaner asked if she should come back tomorrow, and was told that would be fine. The following day when the home help arrived at the back door it was still locked and the bathroom light still on. The question was asked again if the old lady was OK and the answer came again that she was in the bath. The cleaner went away a bit bothered and after due thought rang me to ask if I could come and see what was happening. We broke into the house to find that the poor old girl had been stuck in the bath for at least two days. She had kept warm by topping the bath up with hot water but had forgotten to mention that she could not get out of it. Apart from her skin being waterlogged, she had come to no harm.

Having described my breaking and entering, the same treatment was served up to us. Our surgeries were broken into on three occasions during my time in the practice, once in the old building and twice in the new. For the first break-in at our original surgery, the thieves must have had a child to put through a small upper window flap that had been left open, who then opened a bigger window to let in the robbers. A mess made, but nothing valuable lost.

The second break-in took place shortly after we had moved into our new building. The place had been ransacked, every drawer opened, every record thrown out of their racks; the whole place was a vast mess. Our invaluable wives as well as all the off duty staff turned up to restore some kind of order while we managed to run our surgeries. Nothing significant was taken, as none of us kept scheduled drugs or cash in the place. Several boxes of phials for blood tests were removed, presumably in the mistaken belief that they were vials for injections. Months later they were found by a shooting party, dumped in a nearby wood. The prescription pads that were taken could have been a problem. We were instructed to sign all our prescriptions from then on in red ink, and all chemists in Devon were asked to query any script from us not signed with red ink. A week later two boys were arrested in Plymouth for presenting one of our prescriptions to a chemist, for a scheduled drug, signed with blue ink. The writing on it was even worse than any doctor's. They stated that they had bought the prescription blank from a man that they had met in a pub, and had nothing to do with the break-in.

The third break-in caused severe damage to part of the building. The thieves had got onto the roof and removed some tiles. From the roof space they had stamped through the ceiling of one of the consulting rooms and got in that way. Once in the room, on opening the door to the corridor, we assumed that they had seen the fire sensor and thinking it was part of an alarm system progressed no further and took nothing, but left a great deal of repair work to be done. We put in an alarm system after that.

This may hurt a little...

Things that go wrong

We all make mistakes, errors of judgement, and have human failings and gaps in knowledge. Our practice expected each of us to go away to attend a week's refresher course every year, and we attended many evening lectures from local specialists and of course read the medical journals. It was said that in the 1990s the half-life of medical knowledge was ten years; i.e. half of what we had been doing ten years ago was probably not appropriate now. Keeping up to date required discipline and part of the value of a partnership was that one could also benefit from the knowledge of the others. We always had a Monday lunch of bread, cheese and coffee in the surgery, where we would often invite other professionals such as the local dentists, pharmacists, health visitors and district nurses so we could pick their brains and give them our views on what was happening. The trainees would also be asked on occasions to present cases to us so as to help keep us up to date with the changes in knowledge that were happening.

On several occasions we even had the local MPs in to give him and her advice and to lobby for what changes we felt were needed. Twice the MPs asked to come to lunch so that they could ask our opinion on subjects that they had numerous complaints about, such as disabled parking badges.

Naturally over my time in the practice I have made several errors in judgement that were always a source of regret. I had been seeing the late middle aged wife of an old soldier who had been in the parachute regiment during the war and had survived Arnhem, and for both of whom I had the greatest respect. For a number of years I used to see her, about every six months or so, when she would come in looking well but complaining of an abdominal pain. I would do a careful examination of her abdomen, never finding anything wrong, would reassure her that all was well, and she left content until I saw her again a few months later. She had had shingles in that area some years before and we put the pain down to a post-herpetic neuralgia. One winter evening when the surgery was running extremely late she came in with the familiar story. I was dismissive, did not examine her, and told her to come back if the pain was not better in the usual two weeks. I saw nothing of her for a month and when she came back, for the first time since I had known her, she looked ill. On internally examining her I found a large cancerous tumour in her pelvis. She was referred to hospital and the tumour excised. However, she needed chemotherapy to deal with the secondary spread of the cancer and after several months died in the district hospital, having refused, when she was dying, to come into the local hospital to be under my care.

Her husband, naturally, was furious with me and had no problem in telling me so. I had been dismissive towards her that evening, for which there was no excuse. It was upsetting that two people who I had greatly valued were either dead or furious with me. I felt thoroughly guilty so took to calling in on the widower at his home, after my Tuesday evening surgery, to give him the chance to get his feelings off his chest, an opportunity which he certainly took. I took care never to make any futile excuses for my negligence, such as I was tired after a long day, or that most of her previous attendances had been trivial. He was not only angry with me, but with the hospital that had seen her in London, because they had once lost her medical records, and he would not go to their previous local pub because the bereavement card that they had sent him had been rather too small.

The man was angry with the world as well as with me. My weekly expiation of my guilt was worthwhile, because after a bit if I waved at him as I passed in the car he started to wave back instead of turning his head away as he used to, and we became friends again. Three years later he remarried and asked me if his new wife could join my list of patients. One evening, shortly after joining my list, she came into the surgery with an undefined abdominal pain. I examined her carefully, found nothing wrong, but lost my nerve and referred her to a surgeon explaining to him my reasons for the referral. Luckily all was well.

On another occasion I was telephoned after midnight by a woman who I knew well. Penny told me that Fred, her husband, had been to greyhound racing and had come back with a bad headache. "Has he been drinking?" I asked. "You know Frederick!" was her answer, so I told her to put him to bed with a couple of paracetamol and a long drink of water and to let me know if he was not better in the morning.

As it happened the next day I was away, and on my return my senior partner told me that he had been called to see Frederick and had had to send him into the local neurosurgical unit with a brain haemorrhage. The advice at that time from the Medical Defence Union was never to say sorry as you would be admitting guilt. This is and was poor advice and gives the impression that you do not care about your mistakes. I went straight round to their council house and rang the doorbell. The door opened and when Penny saw who it was she scowled at me. I said that I had come to apologise, that I should have known that they never called unnecessarily. I told her that I had rung the hospital and they had said that he was improving and was not going to need an operation. She immediately smiled and said, "After what I said to you I don't blame you", acknowledging that she had colluded with me in dismissing the call as trivial.

I am certain that honesty with people is the best way; most reasonable people do not expect perfection from doctors but do expect the doctor to take care and to mind about making an error. Similarly I believe in stating that you do not know what is going on, if that is the case, but to say that it does not seem serious, and invite them back if the problem continues or worsens. Adults are well aware if you are prevaricating, and even very young children recognise a phony smile, often bursting into tears if greeted by one. Imagine how it would feel if a stranger suddenly turned towards you in a train with a synthetic grin.

I once had a complaint about my conduct telephoned to the NHS administrators. I was coming to the end of a morning surgery at 1.00pm, I had a patient with me and one more patient to see, when a somewhat aggressive patient arrived demanding to be seen. I agreed to fit him in, and he took his place in the waiting room. I finished my present consultation and as I called the next patient, the newcomer jumped to his feet and demanded to be seen first. As it happened the man that I had just called was in danger of missing his bus if delayed so the aggressive bloke was asked to wait until I had finished with the first man. He then told the receptionist that if he was not allowed to jump the queue he would go home and demand a visit. He was told that this would not be answered and to be patient and wait his turn.

He left the surgery and telephoned soon after (he lived close by) demanding a visit. I spoke to him, told him that I would wait if he returned to the surgery but on no account would I visit. I asked the receptionist to make contemporaneous notes about the incident as I was sure that, on the man's past form, there would be an official complaint. Sure enough, within minutes an NHS administrator was on the phone suggesting that the easiest thing to do would be to do the visit that he had asked for. I replied that if I did the visit I would probably kill him, but I would wait at the surgery for a further length of time to see if he came back. Shortly after this a doctor from a neighbouring practice rang to say that he had been asked to visit the man, and asked what the fuss was about. Having heard what had happened he too refused to visit. In the end the official complaint was dismissed as groundless and in fact the man's need for an urgent consultation turned out to be an attack of mild diarrhoea, which stopped without any treatment.

The extra time lost and emotion caused by that kind of unreasonable behaviour takes a toll, and what should have been an enjoyable day's work was overshadowed by the actions of a self-centred individual. Thankfully this kind of incident was extremely rare in our part of the world.

I was asked to care for an old widow who in her advanced years had come down to spend the rest of her life with her nephew and his wife. He was a rather dour character that I did not know well. I was asked to see the old lady one afternoon because, as she confided to me, that she thought that her nephew was trying to poison her. There was absolutely no evidence for this suspicion and after a careful examination I assured her that she was in fine health and in no danger and that she was not being poisoned. She then told me that she was unhappy in the house and wanted to buy a cottage and move in there as she could afford it because she had over a thousand pounds in the Post Office bank. I pointed out that this would not pay for a cottage these days. She told me that one could buy a perfectly good cottage for £50 and as I was a doctor I knew nothing about house prices, and she then asked me to get a solicitor for her to discuss the matter with. She was so set on this course that I agreed to ask a solicitor to call. As I left her room her nephew stopped me and forbade me to get her a lawyer. He must have been listening at the keyhole and the fragments of the conversation that he had heard must have made him think that I was getting her to change her will in my favour. He was pretty abusive and I dug my heels in and said that if she wanted me to get a lawyer I would do so, whatever he said.

Two days later I received in the post an anonymous card with the post mark of that village on it. It read, "As you sow, so you shall reap, you don't think so now but you will soon find out, you pig." Not too awful but unpleasant to get through the post. We had a police station in the town at the time and I went to see the sergeant, a wise old copper. I told him that I was sure it was from the nephew and that I did not want to take it further but did not wish to receive any more like it. I left the matter in his hands.

The sergeant later told me how he had sorted it out. He had called at the house and in the presence of the nephew and the nephew's wife said that I had received this card, which he showed them, and said that I thought that it had come from his aunt and could he identify the handwriting. "That would be just the sort of thing that she would do," the nephew replied. His wife then said, "Don't be silly, Reg, you know that she cannot read or write." At that point the man burst into tears and admitted that he had sent the card. The sergeant said that nothing would come of it as long as he never sent another. I never got another.

Once when doing a village branch surgery a breathless man arrived saying, "Thank goodness you're here, my neighbouring farmer has just had an accident with a chainsaw." Luckily this good guy had been in a field close to where the farmer was trimming an overgrown hedge with a chainsaw. He heard the farmer cry out and knowing that I was doing a surgery in the village came rushing for help. The unfortunate farmer had trimmed a springy sapling which fell down the far side of the hedge and then had bounced back, knocking him down onto his back with the saw falling, still working, across his right thigh. It was a nasty mess but there was no bone damage. I was able to use a shell dressing which I had purloined from my army days, knowing that it might come in useful some time, and it certainly was. An ambulance took him to the nearest large accident unit to patch him up and he made an excellent recovery.

I am not happy with the recent introduction of initiatives such as NHS Direct, walk-in clinics and anything that loosens the bonds between the patient and their general practitioner. This was why, though in partnership, we still kept our own list of patients so that a relationship between the individual doctor and his patient could build up. This becomes particularly important when your patients are reaching the end of their days.

If practically possible being at home is the ideal place to be at the end of one's life. So many recently bereaved spouses have told me how they wished that their partner had been at home when they had died and so many feel guilty at having let the dying patient be admitted to hospital towards the end of their life, often when there was little practical choice in the matter. Many times I would leave the house of a terminally ill patient feeling that I had not achieved much for them, to be later told that, "He always feels better when you have been." Reassurance and the knowledge that you matter to your doctor is hard to quantify, but I feel that it does matter and does make a difference.

Following the research and lead of Dame Cicely Saunders at St Christopher's Hospice, pain control has been better understood and much improved and in most cases, can and should be managed competently by GPs with, if needed, the excellent back-up of the hospice movement and their nurses. I found that successful management of the care of the dying could be very satisfying if a good peaceful death at home was achieved. As for euthanasia, the thought of the doctor becoming a state sponsored executioner fills me with horror. Relatives used to say things like, "Doc, if I ever get ill like Dad, I hope that you will put me down," but if the time came when it was their turn to be moribund I never had even one person ask to be "put down" and I often had the feeling that they hoped that I had forgotten the much earlier conversation.

The new contract negotiated between the BMA and the government in the nineties of the last century changed the responsibility of the GP from having twenty four hour responsibility for his patients three hundred and sixty five days a year. It means that GPs are able to choose to do no night or weekend work, and which also meant no Saturday morning surgeries. This has led to various unconsidered consequences. There is now no need for your GP to live in the town or village in which they work. They can just turn up at the right time, do the work that is needed and go home miles away at the end of the day. The quality of medicine is still practiced to a high standard, but the personal touch gets diluted, as "your" doctor is a less familiar figure. Emergencies at nights and weekends are catered for by doctors that the patients do not know, and who do not know the patients, so errors in judgement are likely to more prevalent and more patients end up in queues in A and E departments.

After I had been in the practice for a while I was asked by the local nursing school to lecture twice a year to post-graduate nurses and the occasional GP refresher course on care of the dying, and I always reinforced the message that if a patient wanted to know what was happening to them, the truth was the only answer. If a woman comes to the surgery with a lump in her breast common sense tells one that she is frightened that it is a cancer. In those circumstances, after examining her, I would say that it might well not be cancerous, but we will consider it a cancer until we prove that it is not. Acknowledging the "C" word clears the decks and an honest consultation follows. The most rewarding event is to find a breast cyst, where one can put a needle into the cyst, draw out the fluid and "hey presto" the lump has disappeared. A very relieved and happy woman then leaves the consulting room.

There were always a few, very few, patients who, when invited to ask if they wanted any more knowledge about the situation and their future, would look you straight in the eye and say that they did not wish to know anything more.

It is not only doctors who at times get unpopular with the patients. One Sunday morning I was called to the small casualty department at our cottage hospital as a four-year-old-girl had been brought in by her father with a nasty infection in the lobe of her left ear. What had happened was that her grandmother, the father's mother-in-law, in spite of his stated instruction that she was not to have the child's ears pierced at that age, had taken her to a body piercer. Grannie had paid for the child to have her ears pierced and "gold" studs put in. The following morning one of the studs had sunk into the fleshy lobe of the child's ear and had become infected. The ear was red and swollen and oozing pus, the stud was buried and out of sight. I could not use a local with the infection present so had to dig it out without pain relief. It did not take long, but the poor child's screams further inflamed her father's fury, and the promised vengeance to be meted out to his mother-in-law as soon as he left the hospital sounded dire. Years later the girl became one of our receptionists at the surgery and could remember the whole episode. She had eventually, but not until the age of eighteen, plucked up the courage to have her ears pierced again.

A lovely young wife had been delivered of a beautiful healthy first baby some two months before. One morning she arrived at the surgery with the babe. She told me that she thought that the new arrival was blind. Indeed she was correct, and I confirmed the bad news. Her response was to give the little girl a kiss and say, "Never mind darling, Mummy loves you just as much." Enough to make one want to weep.

One of the most alarming and distressing events in my medical life occurred one night after a normal home delivery of a young woman's second child at her somewhat isolated house. The woman had recently moved down to Devon and joined my list when she was about twelve weeks pregnant. She appeared thoroughly healthy and very robust, the only unusual feature of hers a nine square inch skin graft scar over her right biceps, not irregularly shaped as it would be if it had been a burn scar that had been grafted, but neatly rectangular in shape. I had not yet received her past records, but she told me that a mole had been removed from there, a couple of years before. As she was pregnant any X-ray was inadvisable. It seemed likely that a malignant melanoma had been excised widely and deeply and the area then grafted. The pregnancy proceeded absolutely normally with her in apparent good health. When the pregnancy came to term she went into labour naturally and, as planned, had the home delivery. The night that she went into labour the district midwife called me as she made progress and I attended when she became ready to push. As with most second pregnancies the labour was efficient and trouble free and we were soon enjoying the healthy new arrival.

However, within a few minutes of the afterbirth being safely delivered, the young mother suddenly became intensely breathless and in acute distress. There was no alternative but to call an ambulance and arrange for her immediate admission to an acute medical ward. Her poor husband had no choice but to stay at home, because of the sleeping older child, while the new mother went off in the ambulance accompanied by the midwife and the new baby. The poor woman died later the next day, and at a subsequent post mortem it was found that her lungs were full of secondary tumour from the original melanoma. There had been no evidence of illness during her pregnancy or during her labour until after the placenta had been delivered, when her horrifying struggle to breathe started. I have never before seen, and hope never to see again, such a joyful moment turn so suddenly into an unforeseen and irremediable tragedy. Presumably the change in her circulation's dynamics after the delivery triggered the dramatic collapse.

We do not often get heavy snow in the West Country, and on only two occasions in my thirty years of practice here was there enough snow to totally disrupt the day's work. I had seen a four-year-old-girl in the surgery the day before the heavy snowfall. She was suffering from an acute attack of diarrhoea and vomiting. Her farming parents were both competent individuals so I gave them advice on how to manage the situation and she returned with them to her distant farm home. The following morning her mother rang to say that her condition had worsened and could I visit. There had been a heavy snowfall that night with large drifts blocking the roads. I trudged some two miles through the snow to a crossroads, where the child's uncle, driving a tractor, met me and was able to deliver me to within quarter of a mile of their farm. Once there it was obvious that she needed intravenous fluids so a helicopter was organised to fly her to the district hospital where she recovered within a day or two. I re-joined her uncle on the tractor and he took me on to a village which the district nurse could not get to where I gave the needed injections on the nurse's behalf, and then walked the three miles back home. I was exhausted by the time that I reached my home; ploughing through the deep snow was tiring.

On the other winter occasion when a blizzard was blowing, I was asked to visit a man in a village, only a mile and a half away, who sounded as if he was having a heart attack. It was a pitch black evening with driving snow so I decided it would be safer if I was accompanied by my elder son who was then a robust fifteen-year-old. Suitably clad and carrying sticks and my medical bag we made our way to the patient's house where indeed he was having a myocardial infarction. I did what was necessary and he survived. We made our way home, making a mistake on the way back, by trying to take short cut across a field. With the blackness of the night and the driving snow we got totally disorientated and the short cut became a long cut before we found the road again.

One of my partners, before going on holiday, had asked me to keep an eye on a profoundly deaf old man, currently occupying a bed in our cottage hospital, who was suffering from a bad chest. Being so deaf he was almost impossible to have a conversation with. While examining him I noticed that the pupil of his right eye was enlarged compared with his left pupil. This could have been caused by Horner's syndrome, which is due to the right sympathetic nerve chain being interrupted at the level of his first rib. A rare lung cancer at the apex of the lung – a Pancoast tumour – can cause this so I organised a chest X-ray which indeed confirmed the diagnosis. Feeling very clever I asked the local chest physician to come to the hospital to see what, if anything, could be done for the old boy. He duly arrived, looked carefully at the eye and the X-ray and said, "Well done, Jeremy", and the old man, seeing him gazing intently at his eye, said to him, "My eye has always looked like that ever since I had an accident to it when I was about fifteen." I had made the clever diagnosis on totally erroneous grounds, which was embarrassing in the extreme.

Driving down the lanes with grass growing in the middle of the road was a feature of life in our part of Devon but apart from meeting a herd of cows, a flock of sheep or a large tractor, they were usually empty in the winter. During the summer, visitors' cars would often produce a delay as they nervously froze in the narrow lanes on one's approach. One afternoon I was driving down a sunken lane when a dung spreader working in the field above covered my windscreen as if a huge bird had deposited on it, completely blacking me out for a time. It was lucky that it had been ages since I had cleaned the car; it would have been most annoying if I had been driving a nice newly polished clean car.

One of the messiest of jobs that I had to do was on a winter evening when an elderly cowman had fallen from the hayloft of a barn into the midden, and was lying unconscious in ankle deep straw and cow shit amongst the resident bullocks. I did not have my gumboots in the car so after helping retrieve him and dispatch him to hospital everything below my knees was a total mess, as was the inside of the car by the time that I got home.

On another occasion a cheerful rogue, Frankie, who had once been a jockey, ended up his varied career moves as a slaughterman for one of the local butchers. When I first met him he was living with his mother, unmarried elder sister and his brother Peter, who suffered from a severe Down's syndrome. Peter was well into his forties and had never walked. He could not straighten his knees because of contractures and went around on all fours. He was a most amiable character and spent most of his time on his knees on his bed in front of the window engaging with the neighbours as they passed by. His mother was frail and died fairly soon after I started looking after the family, which left his competent elder sister in charge.

Once mum was buried Frank's sister told me that she was not as well as she would like to be, and when I examined her I found that she had a tumour in her abdomen the size of a football. The cancer was inoperable and she died after a short illness. She was another dutiful woman, who had sacrificed her health and life for her family. Frank did not have the ability or inclination to look after Peter who went into care and thrived on the wider world provided than that from his front window. Frankie went to live in an alms room run by a local charity.

He was an amusing, lightweight character known for his good humour and propensity to overload on the booze. One day I was called to the small abattoir at the back of the butcher's shop where a bullock that he had been about to kill had knocked him down and broken his femur. The bullock was still loose in the yard, but seemed peaceful enough so I entered followed by the ambulance men. Frankie was pale and shocked, curled up in one corner of the area. "Well Frankie, at last one got its retaliation in first," I said, somewhat unfeelingly, at which he laughed. Immediately his face went from a ghastly pallor to its usual ruddy hue, and we put him on a stretcher and he left for hospital in much better shape.

Eccentrics and more

There were several eccentrics about the town, who added to the spice of life and, as in most country areas, were tolerated with a degree of affection and vicarious enjoyment and amusement.

My first meeting with Romeo and his family was very early on in my time in the practice. The old patrician partner was still with us and one morning as I was leaving the surgery to start a branch surgery he asked if I could look in on a family as my route went past their house. It was a bit of an ambush as he gave not a hint of the bizarre clan that I was about to meet. Their terraced cottage was in a narrow lane with no parking place near. I parked a little way away, picked up my bag and knocked on the door. I was let into the front room by a very twitchy old man with tattered bandages around both legs. The monolithic figure seated by the fire and looking the shape of a cottage loaf was his wife. As I started the consultation a noise between a grunt and a squeak came from behind the door. I spun round to see another cottage loaf in a Windsor chair looking at me. This was Romeo's sister. Romeo then came in through the door and a strange fragmented conversation started before the immediate problem was identified and as far as I remember sorted out.

Romeo's father did not live for much longer and the remains of the family moved into the town. Mother and daughter going shopping became a sight to see, a female Tweedle-dum being followed by a female Tweedle-dee, both in red duffle coats slowly progressing down the street.

Romeo became a feature of the town, a large noisy man who was quite correctly deemed unfit to look after his not inconsiderable property and money, both of which were handled by the Court of Protection. His nickname of Romeo came from the time that he went around the town with a board tied around his neck with written on it in large clumsy letters "I want a woman".

There were no takers up of this invitation to become Romeo's woman, because he not only looked unattractive but also smelt terrible. Ruth had been a patient in a mental hospital for almost all of her adult life, erroneously so because she was "country simple" rather than insane. After her release from the hospital, she was lodging with and working, as a cleaner, for a woman who was housing several other ex-long term inmates, all of whom had been emptied out of asylums to be sent "home" when the new drug chlorpromazine, "that tamed the mad", came on the market. Needless to say few of the discharged long term patients had homes to go to or families who were prepared to welcome their return, so ended up as bored inmates of several "guest houses" which varied hugely in standard.

Ruth took Romeo up on his offer for the price of two cigarettes. I was asked by Ruth's employer to give her a good talking to for this unappealing act. I did so suggesting that this was not a good idea and anyway it must have been pretty nauseating. She replied, "Yes, it was disgusting, but I did enjoy the two cigarettes."

The staff had a drill for when Romeo attended the surgery. The receptionists would immediately usher him into a small side room away from the other customers, where the doctor would see to him. As soon as he left the premises the girls would come round with much needed deodorising sprays.

Romeo was always demanding that we doctors should petition the Court of Protection to let him have, as he put it, "my affairs back". After a while when none of us, for the best of reasons, would accede to this importuning he took to having lie-down protests in the road in front of the old surgery. Passers-by would look down at him and then up at the surgery windows; they would then behave in one of two different ways. Some, who knew Romeo, would shrug and pass on the other side, whilst the others would walk up to the surgery and tell the receptionist that there was a man collapsed in the road, to be reassured that we knew that and that he was just staging a protest. One damp night, well after the surgery had shut, a man, finding him lying in the road, called an ambulance. The ambulance men knew the score so they just picked him up and put him in through his own front door. Then to cover their backs they rang me to say what had happened and suggested that I should look in on him to see that he was alright.

The house was cold and absolutely disgustingly filthy. Romeo had come to no harm, but I felt a twinge of sympathy for the old rogue as he was soaking wet and all by himself, his mother and sister having died a few years before. I found an electric kettle circa 1920 – it had a wooden handle – nervously plugged it in and made him a pot of tea, after which I swiftly left, with that dreadful feeling that various little beasties had landed on me and were about to start feeding. I raced home for a shower and a change of clothes.

One of my colleagues, who had the privilege to be Romeo's actual doctor, had an exciting call out to see him late one evening. The heroine who ran the telephone exchange at night had rung him up to ask him if he could come and see Romeo, who kept tapping on her window saying that he needed a doctor as he had just received an electric shock when sorting through a litter bin in search of cigarette stubs. My partner duly arrived and after ascertaining that Romeo would live, questioned the source of the supposed electric shock. "You do not get electric shocks from litter bins," he stated with conviction and to demonstrate the fact he put his hand on the bin in question and received a sharp electric shock. The litter bin was fixed to an electric lamppost which had shorted. The story, as told, finished with the pair of them sitting in the gutter side by side, groaning.

I looked after another unusual family consisting of an elderly mother and three late middle aged sons living in the most distant village in our practice. They coped well enough while the old mother was alive but following her death their situation deteriorated fast. I was called there in the middle of one night as the oldest brother had been found in the airing cupboard of their thatched Devon longhouse. He was frantic with delirium tremens, and had in his thrashing about disconnected some of the piping so that there was water spraying everywhere. They lived opposite the village pub and I had not cottoned on to the fact that he was a cider alcoholic, as my visiting to their house had always been on behalf of his old mother. When eventually he came out of hospital I was able to get the publican to refuse to serve him cider and as he never left the village and drank no other alcohol that problem was easily solved.

The middle brother was a simple schizophrenic and no threat to anyone. Though he had a most exciting life, most often very up to date with what was going on in the big wide world. One day, at the time of the Mexico Olympics, he became a multiple Olympic medal winner, proudly giving me a lap by lap and a yard by yard description of all the races that he had just won. During the Vietnam War things got even more exciting. One day when I called in to check on the three old boys I asked him how things were. "I have had a terrible day," he said, "rolling around all morning on the floor of a B12 bomber with a bullet in my guts." Then brushing his sleeves furiously, he said, "And all this bloody radioactivity."

After their mother had died, the three men seemed to exist on nothing but little chocolate covered Swiss rolls and Penguin biscuits. These were always lined up in neatly arranged rows on their kitchen windowsill. At about that time the NHS were starting to introduce the community psychiatric nurses and we were allotted an absolute gem. She took over their domestic arrangements, organising a weekly box of groceries for them, and kept a much needed and much appreciated motherly eye on them. The introduction of these nurses to practices was a huge advance in care by the NHS, as before they were introduced, the vulnerable in society had very little support to help them manage their disordered lives.

A robust and good humoured builder, who never seemed put out about anything, lived with his family in a terraced house in one of our town's streets. He was upset about a developing feud with the old lady who lived next door. She kept coming round to his house and on several occasions complained that he was making loud unpleasant comments about her behind her back. These remarks she claimed that she could hear through the wall between the two houses. This was patently unlikely both physically, but mostly because if he ever wanted to make a comment about someone it was never behind their back and was always good humoured and often very funny. I called in on the old lady to discuss the matter, to find that the voices that she was hearing were obviously hallucinatory and that she was suffering from simple schizophrenia. Once I started treating her, the voices disappeared and so did the aggro, but he never felt happy again with her as a neighbour, and moved house.

Paranoid schizophrenia was a much more difficult a problem to deal with. The usual age of onset is late teens, typically the age when one might be at university and in my experience mostly in males. One very large, physically intimidating, recently graduated electrical engineer, typically started his illness just as he was starting his first employment, having graduated very well from his university. He informed me, with his face a few inches away from mine, that he could "stop time and finish me off just like that" with a click of his fingers. In fact he offered no resistance to my suggestion that he needed hospital care, and though he became rational again, with sustained treatment, he never recovered well enough to hold down a job again.

Equally alarming was a night call to a remote thatched farmhouse where the son of the house was standing on his bed and in the process of tearing a hole in the ceiling above. He was a strapping lad who would easily carry a hundredweight hay bale in each hand; as one passed in the car and waved at him he would casually wave one of the bales at one in return. A frisson of anxiety was always present in these circumstances as one's vulnerability is so marked. The lad said that he was receiving messages from the local pub to break out of the house via the roof. Happily he took my advice and went off to hospital like a lamb, as a voluntary patient, but, alas, never regained his former health or personality and died at a young age.

I was driving down to Plymouth one early afternoon off to take the final oral part of the RYA Offshore Skipper's exam. It was unfortunate that I happened to be following a car on a winding lane. Just after I had left the town, the car ahead stopped abruptly just round a bend causing me to run into the back of it. I got out and discovered that the driver was one of a partner's paranoid schizophrenic patients. He had decided that I was following him for nefarious purposes and had deliberately caused the accident. When I asked him the reason that he had stopped so suddenly, he replied that I was "just the kind of bastard who would run over a little bird in the road". Luckily I managed to hire a car, got to the exam a little late and thankfully passed it.

The most tragic case of sectioning a patient of mine occurred when an eighty-six-year-old man became deluded about his fifty-year-old youngest son, who lived several miles away. The old boy conceived the totally groundless idea that his son was having sexual relations with the old boy's wife, the son's own mother.

Not only that, but he believed that his son was driving around the village mocking his father about it. To retaliate against this perceived taunt he took to binding a large pebble into a long scarf, and then he would stand at the side of the road and swing it at the windscreen of any passing car that he fancied might contain his laughing son. Obviously this was so dangerous that it had to be stopped and reasoning with the poor old man had no effect. I had to section him and the pitiful sight of the old chap raging like King Lear, "I will do such things – what they are yet I know not; but they shall be the terrors of the earth", as he was carried into the ambulance, was very upsetting both for the ambulance men and me, but what choice did we have? The poor old fellow died three days later in the mental hospital.

Fred, a widower who lived alone, provided some excitement. He had always been the kind of man who imagined that women fancied him; when he got the idea that a female was in this frame of mind about him he would be a persistent nuisance, indeed the senior partner once had to shake him off from plaguing his wife, by getting his solicitor to write him a letter. For a short time two years after we had arrived in the town, he started to hang around our house, fancying that my wife fancied him, but was easier to get rid of. Whenever he appeared she always said that they were on the way out, loaded the children into the car and drove away. He soon got the message that she did not fancy him.

My mistake was to refer him and his stiff shoulder to a very attractive Swedish physiotherapist who was working at our cottage hospital. She was a slim blonde who looked very fetching in her physiotherapist's uniform. He took to her like a duck to water and then became totally deluded. One day, carrying his shotgun, he approached a neighbouring farmer, and told the farmer that he knew that the farmer had the lovely physiotherapist locked up in one of his chicken sheds, and that she wanted to get to out to be with Fred. He said that if the farmer did not release her within two hours he would shoot the farmer and rescue the girl. He then marched off home and the farmer rang me. I knew Fred very well, so went round to his house, rang his doorbell and when he opened the door told him not to be such an idiot and give me the gun which he did without a murmur. His delusion was so fixed and potentially dangerous that the only solution was to section him, and off he went complaining mildly to hospital.

The only time that I was ever assaulted by a patient was when I was trying to section a young man who, when he was well, was the most affable of people. He had had his first psychotic breakdown at university and came onto my list when he and his retired parents arrived to live in the area. He was being medicated and able to hold down a job. After a settled year he went on holiday and met an American psychologist in a bar. On hearing the man's profession, he made the mistake of telling him of his diagnosis and quoted me as saying, "My doctor says that, just like a diabetic taking insulin, as long as I take these pills I am as healthy as the next man." "Your doctor is a tool of the capitalist state, stop the pills and liberate yourself," was the reply. Unfortunately he took this advice and our troubles started. He was sacked from his job and his behaviour became a growing problem to his parents, with whom he lived, as well as to the neighbourhood.

The crisis came when I was told by a local farmer about an incident that had happened one night in the road just by the farm. I was visiting the farmer's old mother when as I was leaving the farmer said, "You know that young man who lives up the hill?" "Yes." "He's a bit odd, isn't he?" "Why?" "Well last night he suddenly stopped his car just outside here, went round to the car that was following, opened the door, dragged the driver out, punched him to the ground and drove away."

It became obvious that in his situation he needed to be stabilised in hospital and also that he was not going to agree to be admitted as a voluntary patient. By then the law had changed and to force someone to be admitted to a mental hospital against their will required a social worker to agree in conjunction with a doctor.

The only time that this young man was guaranteed to be at his home was on a Saturday late afternoon. I organised a social worker, and with an ambulance around the corner, plus a police car with a couple of policemen, just in case, to stand by on the next Saturday afternoon. This Saturday happened to be my weekend off, but the job needed doing. The social worker and I rang the doorbell and were shown into the house by his parents, who had been forewarned and agreed about this course of action. I asked the youngster came down from his bedroom, and then told him that I thought that he was very ill and needed to be in hospital. He had been sectioned before whilst at university and understood the process. He asked if he could discuss the matter alone with me in the kitchen, which was disconcerting. However depriving someone of their liberty is such a serious matter so, with alarm bells ringing, I agreed to accompany him to the kitchen. On my way there I debated with myself whether to take off my glasses, decided that could be interpreted as a provocative gesture, so decided to leave them on and to sit down as soon as I got to a chair, reasoning that people do not hit other people when they are sitting down. However I was dealing with the irrational. As soon as we got to the kitchen I immediately sat down on the nearest chair, but without a further word he swung round and hit me on the nose, knocking my glasses off, and the chair with me on it went over backwards onto the floor. I shouted for help in an extremely loud voice and the back-up came in at speed. The unlucky social worker got his cornea scratched and his leather jacket pocket torn off, whilst I had a bleeding nose. The police and the ambulance men all did their bit, and suitably sedated, he went off in the ambulance to hospital while I, shaking like a leaf, went off home. We had a party to go to that evening, which I managed to get to after washing my face and changing my clothes and my blood-stained tie.

Four days later, when at a branch surgery, I was telephoned by one of our receptionists to say that a local newspaper had just rung up to say that a man had recently left their office after stating that he wanted them to announce that he was issuing a death threat against me. I telephoned the hospital to which he had been committed, to find out if he was still there. "No," they said. They had let him go out to a pub for a drink and he had not returned. I was both worried and cross. He knew where I lived so I rang my wife, told her to get the children in and lock all the doors and windows, and if he came down the drive to immediately call the police, and I then continued with the surgery. He was found later asleep in a barn near his home, and was returned to hospital without resisting.

A few weeks later he was discharged from hospital on medication and restored to health. I came across him walking up the hill about a mile from his home, stopped and offered him a lift home. He got into the car and had complete recall of the incident and apologised for hitting me. He then said that giving him that opportunity made him believe that I was on his side. He said that he now trusted me and what was my advice. I responded that he had not been well and that as I had given him the chance to clobber me, I did not hold it against him in the least. We arranged that he would continue with his present medication without missing a single dose, and that if he ever felt that he was losing control he should ring the surgery where he would be seen at once by me, or if I was away by one of my partners. Until he and his parents moved away the bargain held and he never needed a hospital admission again.

Another alarming incident was solved by sectioning, with the help of the police, a young man who had a history of a previous psychotic breakdown, and was threatening his parents' lives. He had them locked into their house having attempted, the night before, to disconnect the gas supply and blow the house up. His father had fortunately prevented this. Father managed to get to the telephone during the next morning and gave a breathless message to the surgery, "Get the doctor here quick". The surgery radio got hold of me on my rounds and I immediately drove round to their house to find the doors locked, but listening at the door I could hear voices inside.

The doorbell was not answered so after due thought I rang the police. The copper who arrived broke the door down and we silently gathered at the foot of the stairs and listened. We could hear the sound of three voices chanting a prayer coming from one of the bedrooms upstairs. On a previous visit to the house a year earlier I was pinned in my car by a very belligerent Alsatian dog until he was grabbed by his master and tied up. There were no signs of the dog so we presumed it was in the room with the house's three other inhabitants. The policeman called his inspector explaining the situation. He duly arrived with a police dog handler and we formed a plan. The inspector was most competent. He had brought with him a riot shield and he planned that he would burst through the bedroom door first and pin the lad to the wall with the shield while the dog handler would follow in and get the dog.

We crept silently up the stairs and waited on the landing. The inspector whispered, "One, two, three, GO" – and in they went. The plan worked a treat. The lad was immediately pinned to the wall and had no chance to do any damage to anyone. His parents scuttled out onto the landing, seeming diminished in size, with the father exclaiming in relief, "What took you so long?" The Alsatian turned out to be a different one from that of my previous encounter and could not have been more pleased to see us and be freed. The boy was put into the police car and driven away to hospital giving me a look of pure hatred as he went.

He was never willing to take any regular medical treatment that would have helped him and once he had been released from hospital continued to be a source of great anxiety to his parents. I would only give him a sick note for a month at a time so he had to come in to see me every month, and always with his father present. Every time that he came to see me he would tell me in detail of his hatred for me and the way that I controlled his life. Once he demanded a letter from me stating that I gave him permission to leave the country, which of course I was happy to do. He was the only patient I ever looked after that really frightened me. Being looked at with unblinking implacable hatred is unnerving. Some time after I had retired one of the partners told me that he had committed suicide.

Night calls

The variety of calls at night could be astonishing, some life-saving and others plainly and annoyingly trivial. Our contract, as for every GP at that time, was to provide medical care for the patients on your list for twenty four hours a day and for every day of the year. You could share the out of hours work with partners, or pay a locum to take over the responsibility, but there was no other alternative available if you wanted to be an NHS sub-contracted General Practitioner. Now the current contract can absolve the doctor from that responsibility, moving your doctor to a much more arm's-length relationship.

There was nothing more upsetting than getting to the village or street in the dark and having difficulty in finding the house. Some houses still have no number or name on them, or the number displayed on them was so small that it could not be read in the dark. I soon learnt, if I did not know the house, to ask the caller to switch on every light possible so they would be easier to find. One awful night I had been called to a house in a new estate that I knew, but which was unnumbered. The solitary man had had a coronary thrombosis and was very ill. I had just called an ambulance when the patient collapsed. I started doing CPR on the man; shortly after, I heard the ambulance going up and down the roads in the estate trying to find the house, knowing that if I stopped he would die. The upshot of the matter was that the unfortunate man died. He probably would have done so anyway, but without the ambulance's arrival it became a certainty.

When the telephone by the bedside rang one's reaction was very much triggered by what time of night it was and if I had just sunk into a deep sleep usually it took me some time to emerge from it. I remember once being actually asleep whilst answering the phone. The husband of the patient needing attention, a retired Brigadier, was on the phone and told me that his wife's tongue had suddenly swollen up and she could not get it back in her mouth. My response was a slurred, "What an extraordinary thing." He replied, "Doctor, I do not think that you understand," and repeated the nature of the problem. My wife meanwhile was hitting me in the ribs with her elbow and telling me to wake up. Eventually I surfaced, to which he said, "That sounds better," and repeated the nature of the problem. She was obviously having an anaphylactic reaction to something. I was at their house within twenty minutes, administered a subcutaneous injection of adrenalin and her tongue shrunk back to its usual proportions and popped back into her mouth. I was duly thanked with an amused reference to my slow response.

When dealing with the delivery of babies in the early hours one could feel very isolated and vulnerable when a problem with the confinement occurred, being all on one's own apart from the midwife and the patient. On one occasion I was dealing with a baby, still in his mother's uterus, whose heartbeat was slowing down and then speeding up alarmingly. These signs meant that the unborn child was in distress. The foetal heart monitor had not been invented which meant keeping a close listening watch with the stethoscope on mum's tummy. The baby was ready to be delivered but needed a helping hand to speed up the process.

I applied the hospital's obstetric forceps but the handles did not come together. Obstetric forceps are made in two halves arranged so that when applied correctly the two handles fit snugly together. This means that the babe's head is safely and correctly cradled between the blades and applying pressure to deliver the child will do the babe no damage. On this occasion I could not get the handles to come together properly. I removed them and reapplied them a couple of times with the same result. By that time the baby's heart rate was all over the place and I knew that the child was in danger of dying and would be safer in a cot than in mum's uterus, so I reapplied the forceps without the handles coming together and delivered her with my heart in my mouth as to whether I would be the cause of any brain damage to the child. When she was safely delivered we could see that the application of the forceps was perfect, even though the handles had not come together, and there was no sign of damage to the child. I looked very carefully at the forceps and discovered that they were not a pair. I was horrified, having died a thousand deaths of anxiety as to whether I was going to cause death by doing nothing or causing irrevocable damage to the baby by using badly applied forceps. I asked the midwife to take them down to the hospital administrator that morning and to get a correctly matching set.

The sister midwife rang me later to say that the hospital manager had put the two blades together, held them up to the light and said, "They look alright to me, tell the doctor that he will just have to get on with them." I blew my top after all the last night's stress, so rang him back telling him in no uncertain terms that, if a new pair of forceps were not at the hospital by this evening, I would be ringing the *Daily Mirror* to tell them the story. I do not like having to use threats like that, but after the anxiety and fear of the night I was not going to take no for an answer. Needless to say that evening he telephoned to say that a new, matching pair were now in the labour ward.

Once I was rung up very late at night by an attractive young woman whose husband had recently left her. "Doctor there are a couple of flies flying around in my bedroom and I cannot get to sleep. Could you come and help?" My wife hissed at me, "Leave this bed and you are divorced." I calmed the woman down by talking quietly to her and heard no more, and am still married to the same wife.

Another memorable night call was to a house with a toddler who was far from well. It was about 3.00am when I got to their house and it was obvious that the infant had a bacterial meningitis and needed an urgent hospital admission. The quickest way to accomplish this was for me to immediately drive him and his mother to hospital, rather than wait for an ambulance to arrive, so mother and child were loaded into the back of my car and I set off at speed towards the main hospital. This was before the 70mph speed limit had been introduced, and I had a fast car. I was doing 100mph down a long straight road, and about to tell the mother that there could be no faster way to get to the hospital when headlights came into view in my rear mirror and we were overtaken as if we were standing still. We got to the hospital safely and in time for the boy to recover with no permanent damage done.

Amongst the families that I looked after were a few families who were unable to manage their lives, their finances or care for their children. One of these clans had an abundance of children who were often ill. Social Services had taken the youngest into care but the other four were still at home. I was telephoned well after midnight by their mother who said that one of the boys was breathing in a "funny way". What she described sounded like the air hunger of aspirin poisoning. Yes, she had found her four-year-old son with the aspirin bottle in his hand at about 4.00 pm that afternoon. I raced around to the village where they lived and sure enough the laboured "air hunger" breathing fitted in with aspirin poisoning. I put her and the boy into my car and we raced off to the main hospital, but alas we got there too late and he did not survive, dying about four hours later.

Sadly the little girl who had been in care was returned to that family, normally a cause for joy. I went round to meet the child as soon as Social Services had delivered her back to her home. She was an enchanting, wide awake, outgoing little blond girl sitting up in her pram smiling at all and sundry. I called in three days later to see how she had settled in, to find a bedraggled, dirty, dispirited little waif still in the same dress and still in the same pram. In those three days all the fun had gone out of her, and due to idle neglect and the lack of love. It was heartbreaking.

One really annoying call came in within a minute or two after I had returned from another night visit. I had just got back into bed and was getting comfortable again. It was from a qualified nurse, who should have known better, saying that her son of three years old had woken up screaming, he had not recognised her at first and could I come at once. I suggested that it sounded as if he was having a nightmare, but she insisted that he was ill, so I left my nice warm bed for the second time that night and arrived at their house and rang the doorbell. She opened the door, said, "Yes, it was a nightmare," and shut the door in my face without another word. I felt like kicking the door in and demanding that she at least said thank you. Needless to say, I did nothing of the sort but went back to bed in a fury.

Another qualified nurse, now retired, who also should have known better, once rang me at 3.00am. When I asked what the problem was she cheerfully said that there was no problem, she was just checking on how the night emergency calls worked. I recognised her voice and the following morning told one of my partners the story, naming the culprit. Later that morning he was doing a branch surgery in her village when she turned up there. He told her that I had been not at all happy to have been telephoned at that time of night for such a trivial reason. She had always been a high user of medical time and the benefit of that episode was that she did not dare face me in the surgery for several weeks.

I was once called out in the early hours by the husband of a middle aged woman who had sent him out to the telephone telling him to call the doctor at once. When I got to the house and asked what the problem was I was told that there was no problem, but she had had a feeling that there might be one soon so she wanted to be checked over just in case.

There were compensations, living in the part of the world that we did, in that in the early summer mornings the countryside looked superb and in compensation often a fox, deer or a badger would be crossing the lane to cheer one up. In the darkness the headlights of the car would often show the reflected glow of the eyes of hunting domestic cats in the hedgerows. How there are any hedge nesting birds left seems a miracle. One night, cresting a hill during a violent thunderstorm, the lightning was reflected into my eyes off the shiny wet road so brightly that I was unable to see for a few seconds. It must be a better way of life than practising in a city, though one does spends much more time in the car than a city doctor would.

Another bucolic hazard occurred when I was halted in my urgent journey to a farm, where an experienced mother had just had a precipitate delivery of a baby daughter. My rapid dash to restore order came to a sudden halt when I was obstructed by a sow and some score of her piglets occupying a crossroads. It delayed me a treat, but no harm came to mother or baby or the sow and piglets.

A furious neighbouring doctor once told me "that some silly woman had telephoned him at 1.00am on that early Monday morning." He told me that she had been reading the *Sunday Times* in bed and had come across an article headed "Chloramphenicol the killer drug". This doctor had just prescribed that antibiotic in the form of eyedrops for her daughter's conjunctivitis. She had panicked and telephoned him at that hour of the night to ask if the eyedrops that he had prescribed for her daughter were safe to continue using tomorrow morning.

As it happened, I was talking to the Lady's Circle in that same town a week or two later with the subject being "How to Treat Your Doctor". The idea was to coach these women on the best approach when asking for a visit or advice. For instance, ringing up at 6.00pm and saying, "My little boy has been unwell these last three days and it is time that something is done about it," goes down less well than saying, "My little boy has been unwell for three days and suddenly has got worse, could you possibly call and see him?"

Anyhow after the talk as usual questions came from the audience. A member of the audience told me that she had been reading the *Sunday Times* in bed late the other Sunday evening and came across this article about the antibiotic in her daughter's eyedrops being dangerous when taken orally. She had immediately rung her doctor to ask if it was safe to continue the drops. Her question was, "Would Dr X have minded that I rang him about this in the middle of the night?" I said, tongue in cheek, that knowing Dr X as I did, I was sure that he would have taken it in his stride.

In the same neighbouring town another of the doctors was woken by the doorbell at 2.00am one morning. Putting on his dressing gown he went downstairs, and opened the door to find one of his patients on the doorstep. "I just happened to be passing doctor and wondered if you would mind looking at this boil that I have on my arm." This particular doctor, who had a well-deserved reputation for kindness and tolerance, looked at the boil, gave advice and a prescription for an antibiotic, and went back to bed, while the patient also went home to bed satisfied. The doctor thought about it and decided on a gentle revenge; the next time he was out at the local obstetric unit at an inconvenient hour of the night, he would call at that patient's house and ask him how the boil was. Sure enough he was returning at 2.00am from delivering a baby a day or two later and decided to have his revenge. He parked the car outside the man's house and rang the doorbell. The bleary-eyed pyjama-clad patient opened the door. The doctor opened the conversation with, "I just happened to be passing so I thought that I would look in to see how your boil was getting on." The rejoinder was unexpected. "Doctor, how wonderful you are, what a kind man you are. Mabel, get up at once. The doctor is here, you must make him a cup of tea." So the poor guy was totally disarmed and had to spend twenty minutes longer out of bed drinking his cup of gratefully given tea.

Trying to get one over a patient is not usually a successful exercise. A bothersome cider alcoholic came to see me on a Monday morning stating unequivocally that he had swallowed both full sets of his false teeth. This was patently impossible and he had probably vomited them into a ditch somewhere. He would only be pacified by me arranging an X-ray of his abdomen, though I knew that even if he had managed to swallow his plastic false teeth, with the then X-ray techniques, that they would not show up on simple X-rays. I fixed this up, but my deceit was ruined by the radiologist telling him that I should have known that his false teeth would not show up on the X-ray.

A self-inflicted night call came about on a totally miserable wet and windswept, cold January night. The kind of night that being dozy and snuggling warmly under the bedclothes is never more appealing. I had got in at about 11.00pm having delivered a baby boy in a cottage in our most distant village. The labour had been trouble free and the delivery complicated only by having to speed up the delivery of the babe's head with an episiotomy. This I had carefully repaired with stitches, I then examined the healthy child, enjoyed the delight and relief of the new parents, drank a cup of tea with them, and had departed home for another hot drink and bed. Just as I was dozing off, reviewing the evening's work, I was struck with a dreadful doubt. As was my usual practice, before starting the repair, I had put a swab high into the mother's vagina to mop up any blood that might have seeped down and stopped one seeing the wound clearly, which is necessary if a good repair is to be done. I could not recall having removed it. I wrestled with the thought one way and the other. "I always remove it. I could not possibly have left it in," but, argue with myself as long as I liked, I knew that, for my peace of mind, I would have to go back and check. I got up, dressed and drove back to the cottage and rang the doorbell. Luckily they had not settled down for the night though they were surprised at my arrival. I explained that I had come to check that I had not left a swab in. I examined her and to my intense relief, there was no swab. Back home again and into bed to sleep with a great sense of relief and a clear conscience.

One of the most annoying calls occurred one filthy wet night. I was telephoned up by a lay preacher from his comfortable warm bed, who said that he had just been telephoned by a "poor benighted soul" who he thought had need of a doctor. He then gave the name of a very confused woman who we knew well. She would ring random telephone numbers at any time of day and often at night. Her random calls were so frequent and so fatuous that the electricity board, water board and many other utilities would no longer accept any of her calls.

However I duly dressed and drove to her cottage, which lay the other side of a small stream, now well in spate. The night was pitch black and sheeting down with rain. After I had crossed the little bridge into her garden, I trod into an overflowing flower bed with my right shoe, filling it with muddy water. When I got to her lit conservatory I could see in through the glass and there she was, looking fit and well and talking on the phone. I hammered on the glass again and again, failing to attract her attention. I went back down the path, this time filling my left shoe with mud and water in the identical place where the path curved and where I had drowned my right shoe on the way in. Getting to the car I called up Ann on the radio and explained what was happening and asked her to telephone the old lady to say that I was outside. A thoughtless request as when she tried to phone the line was constantly engaged. I went back up the path again; this time I managed to avoid treading in the mud soaked flower bed, for one more fruitless attempt to let the old bird know that I was there. No luck, so home to bed soaking wet and muttering under my breath.

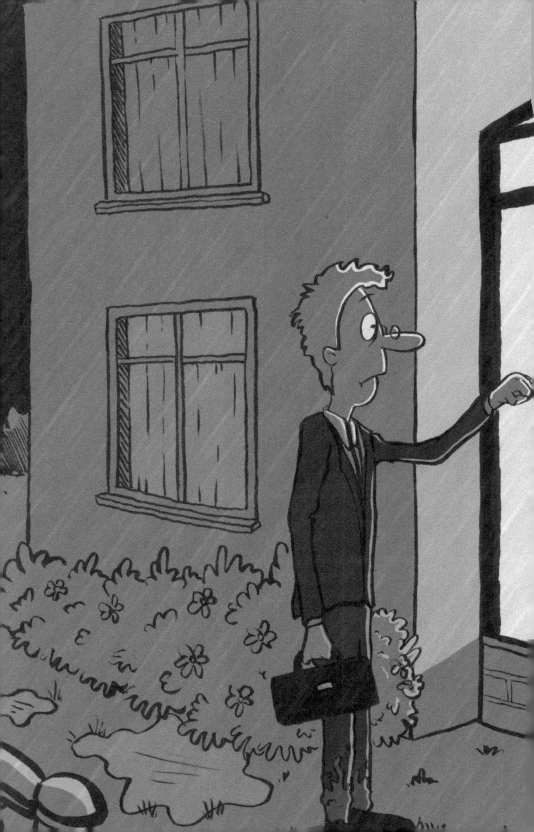

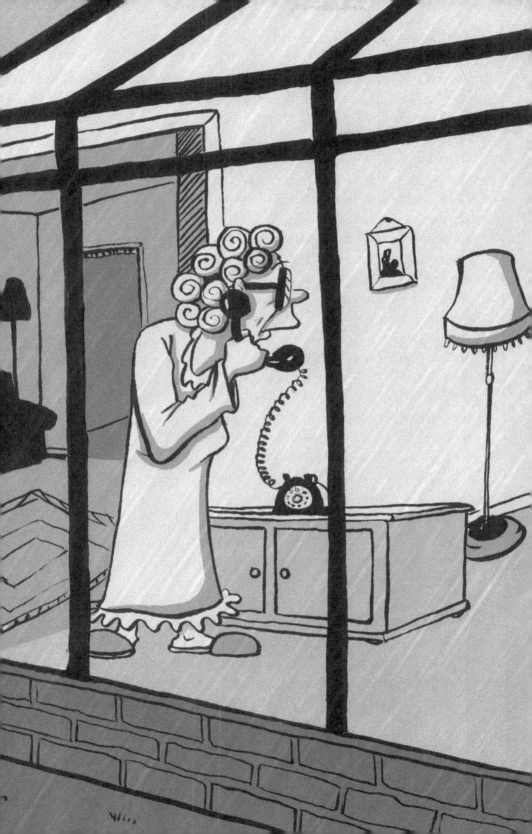

I resisted the temptation to telephone the preacher to wake him up and tell him that the old lady was fit and well.

Several late evening calls would come from various police stations around the district where an urbane sergeant would say, "We have one of your patients here, Doc. He has asked for you to come and take the blood test for alcohol as he does not fancy the local police surgeon sticking a needle in him." I would then ask if I could speak to their male victim; never to my recollection was it a female asking for my attendance. The voice of the miscreant would then come on the phone oozing with unctuous bonhomie and charm: "'Ullo Squire – these plods say that I am drunk in charge of a car, could you come and take my blood for the test?" A well-known, playing for time, manoeuvre. I would politely say, "No. Sorry but I am on call for the whole practice and cannot drive miles out of the area in case there is an emergency here." Once because the offender was a patient of mine with major psychiatric problems I did go to the police station in the next door town. The bloke was indisputably drunk and unfit to drive. I told him so as I took his blood. He then said that he would get a Yorkshire Jewish lawyer to defend him as they were the best lawyers in the world. "These ignorant country coppers would not know what had hit them." All this said at the top of his voice, in front of the police. Subsequently in spite of legal help from a local lawyer, neither Jewish or a Yorkshire man, he did not get off his inevitable ban.

Once I was also called on by an incorrigible patient of mine for whom I had an inexplicable fondness, who asked if I could come to court and state, under oath, that his crime of breaking into his gas meter was due to "an irresistible impulse" that he could not have been expected to resist. I told him that I could not do that and we still remained friends.

The roving drug addicts on the search for extra drugs would occasionally turn up, usually on a Saturday morning with some story such as that he had been looking over the side of a bridge when their supply of drugs had inadvertently fallen into the river and could I supply a replacement prescription. My answer was always "No". If one got a name for being a soft touch with these gentlemen word went round that you were easy meat and you got more harassed. One day, having refused this request in the surgery, when I went up to the cottage hospital, who should I find there but the same guy waiting to try it on with the hospital doctor. He was bitterly disappointed to find that the hospital doctor was the same miserable character who had refused his first request. When I left the hospital, after my rounds, I was mightily relieved to find that my car's tyres had not been let down.

This may hurt a little...

Dying

I am sure that human beings can by sheer willpower hasten their own deaths and also postpone the event until they feel free to let go. I can give several examples of both scenarios.

A very practical efficient businesswoman was dying from a terminal cancer at our cottage hospital. In the same hospital her husband, who had had a major stroke, and had never recovered consciousness, was also dying. She told me that she had to die after her husband did, as she had all the family money, earned by her hard work in her little shop, whilst he had never earned much or saved much as a school caretaker. She pointed out that in her will she was leaving her estate to her husband so she thought, erroneously, that if she died first there would be estate duty raised on her estate and then taxed again when her husband died. If he died first she said that estate duty would only have to be paid on her estate as he was leaving her nothing. Sure enough, she hung on until he died and then within four hours of that event she let herself die.

A middle aged farmer was farming a very small holding, left to him by his parents who had died four years before. He had never managed to find himself a bride in spite of having been a member of the Young Farmers, the usual way of finding a spouse for the farming community at that time. He was isolated, lonely and making very little money as the scale of the farm meant that subsistence level farming was all that was possible for him. He told me one day that the next time that he was ill he was going to die. A few months later he caught a cold, not a particularly severe one, but as he lived alone, he fixed up with a neighbour to look after his six cows and I took him into our small hospital to make sure that he was looked after and fed properly until he recovered. He got more and more unwell, without any apparent reason that

I could discern for why his condition should be deteriorating. Bewildered, I transferred him to the district general hospital where he gently died without any discernible pathological cause for his death, other than that, presumably, he was wanting to die.

Another determined elderly widow was suffering from a terminal cancer, but was not yet moribund. Her pain was well controlled with oral morphine and there seemed no reason to believe that her death was imminent. She told me one evening that she was going to die that night as it would be very convenient as her two much travelled sons were at the time nearby and her death now would inconvenience them the least. I reassured her that I did not visualise her dying that night, but counted her morphine pills just in case she might try to overdose herself. The following morning when I came to see her she was extremely cross to be alive. "When I set out to achieve something I always succeed," she stated firmly. I counted her morphine tablets again and the numbers showed that she had not tried to overdose herself. I told her that she was far from dying and that she would probably be disappointed again tomorrow. The next morning she was dead. I counted her pills again and she had not taken an overdose. I am certain that she had died from a determination to die.

I can recall occasions such as when a distant much loved son or daughter is hurrying to get back to see mother before she dies and a peaceful death takes place within a few hours of the child's arrival to bid farewell. Also once when the patient hung on until a much wanted grandchild was safely delivered, having told me that she would wait to die until she heard that news.

Suicides

There was a spate of suicides one November, all by hanging, and all of them tragic. If one was treating the patient at the time I was always left with a guilty feeling that I should have foreseen the event and somehow done more to prevent the act.

I remember well a very nice kind and thoughtful man who had been widowed, for almost a year, after caring wonderfully well for a dying wife over several months. He had nothing to reproach himself for as his care and commitment to her was second to none. After her death he developed a severe clinical depression. His brothers and a sister kept a good eye on him, often having him living with one or other of them, and he was actually staying with his eldest brother on the day that I last saw him alive. His brother had driven him into the surgery, and came in with him to see me. The widower seemed much more his old self that day, not as flat in mood as he had been previously. I commented on this and he said that he had been feeling much better recently, and his brother sitting behind him nodded and gave me the thumbs up sign. He then told me that he was going on to stay with his sister tonight as she needed her potato patch digging and the potatoes bagging, which he would be doing for her tomorrow.

The following afternoon his sister rang me to say that she had found him dead, hanging in her garden shed. All the potatoes had been dug and were neatly bagged up. When I got there he was hanging from a low beam in the garden shed with his knees almost touching the floor. He could have stood up at any time if he had chosen to, which would have prevented his death. I am sure that the reason he had seemed to be improving from his desolation was because he had made a decision that after getting his sister's potatoes sorted out he would end his life. Having made that resolution he felt easier in his mind. However sometimes any small improvement in a depressive illness gives the patient enough recovered drive to be able to take the decisive step and to get on with their suicidal act, from which their previous lack of drive has held them back.

One evening a reassuringly comfortably large police constable rang me to say that he had been called to a house where the householder had been discovered hanging in his garage. When I got to the house it was obvious that the poor chap had been dead for some little while. The garage floor was at a much lower level than the house to which it was adjoined. The connecting door to the garage came in onto a small landing from which the stairs turned at a right angle going down the side of the garage wall down to the garage floor. The poor man had tied the cord with which he used to hang himself at a good distance from the little landing out onto a roof beam and after tying the cord around his neck had jumped from the landing into space. He was suspended some eight feet above the garage floor. As the copper was a more solid build that I was, we agreed that he would be down on the garage floor to do the catching whilst I would reach out to cut the rope and let him down. I managed my part without a problem but the falling corpse knocked the policeman down, who then promptly fainted. Not the most satisfactory or dignified way of coping with the matter.

Another sad suicide was of the hardworking father of a young man who, though born a normal little boy, through a developing congenital abnormality, epiloia, developed an increasing loss of intellect and by the time that I took over his care he was a strapping six foot young man with the mental development of a four-year-old. His five foot tall mother managed him wonderfully well, he did what she told him to do, and there was no problem with the quality of the care provided. He could be quite alarming to be with because he had a large comfort sheet of cloth which he would suck at the corner and then crack it like a whip inches from one's face. Mother would tell him to stop and good as gold he would stop for a time, before forgetting and starting cracking it at one all over again. He was extraordinarily accurate and the cloth never touched me, always stopping an inch or two away. His father, however, could not cope well with the disappointment and the strain of living with the boy and had started drinking cider very heavily. What trigger eventually pushed him into the final action of hanging himself in their garden shed was never apparent.

After his father's death the young man became much more difficult for his tiny mother to handle and out of the blue he suddenly punched her hard in the face leaving her with a black eye and a complete loss of confidence. She became terrified of him, so he ended up having to be institutionalised, which left his poor mother riven with guilt.

One of the saddest botched suicide attempts that I attended was of a young married woman who was suffering from a post-natal depression. She had thrown herself out of an upstairs window onto a paved area and sustained a fractured skull. She recovered her health fully when the depression passed, but was left clumsy with one arm and blind in one eye.

The most grisly successful suicide that I ever attended was of an old man, once a vagrant, who had lodgings in the town. As he had aged he had decided that life on the road was getting too hard and was fixed up with this motherly soul who did her best to make him feel comfortable and welcome. He never really settled down stuck in one place and with increasing despair had cut his own throat with such force that, apart from severing his neck veins and arteries, he had opened up his windpipe. The poor old lady that he lodged with was faced with a dreadful scene of carnage when she took him his evening cocoa.

Shotgun suicides were rare, though there were plenty of legally owned guns in the rural community. I saw only two episodes where a shotgun was used for that purpose. One of my schizophrenic patients had successfully killed himself using a shotgun, whilst the other incident of an attempted suicide using a shotgun was by a farmer's wife. She had a wound that had almost amputated her breast, but fortunately without any of the shot entering her thoracic cage. She came back to full fitness after the wound and her mind had healed.

I wish that there was a better name for clinical depression than "depression". It might be better understood if it had a different label. Feeling depressed is something that anyone can feel at appropriate times and for recognisable and understandable reasons such as bereavement or a disappointment in love. This normal type of depression usually sorts itself out over given time and is never helped by anti-depressant drugs, though occasionally it can move on to become an endogenous depression.

A full blown clinical depression is a severe debilitating illness, often as part of a bipolar syndrome, alternating with times of exhilaration leading on to hypomania and even to mania itself, as suffered by the previously mentioned vicar's wife. It carries with it a significant mortality rate. Often it strikes when the life and circumstances of the victim are fine, making an obvious cause inexplicable. Perhaps with a different name this dreadful illness would be regarded with more understanding by the general public. "Get a grip of yourself", "Pull yourself together" and "Cheer up" are such inappropriate comments to a sufferer of a clinical depression. There are successful treatments available if the illness is recognised and the patient can be persuaded that he or she is worthy of treatment.

On occasions one had what might be termed "gesture" attempted suicides taking place, scratches across wrists, aspirin overdoses being taken prior to a telephone call saying what the person had done and almost always in good time for remedial action to be taken. These could be termed "cries for help" or actions of the "I'll show him (or her) what it means to me" type of behaviour. Occasionally these would succeed often through misjudgement, and even more so when paracetamol and alcohol are used instead of the more easily recoverable from aspirin, which it has largely replaced in the bathroom cupboard.

It was with mixed feelings that I retired shortly after my sixtieth birthday; I was tired out and at that age one did not recover from being woken at night in the way that one had done when in one's thirties and forties. I knew that I would miss my patients, my colleagues and the staff when I left. The town gave me a super send off when I retired after over thirty years in the practice. Unlike my predecessor I was not given a television set, but many of my old patients subscribed to a fund for me and many gave me individual presents often associated with sailing, as they knew that Ann and I were planning to sail across the Atlantic. Pilot books, barometers, paintings, empty photo albums, a camera and lots else were given to me. I was given lovely farewell severance parties, with customised cakes, in some of the villages where I had done branch surgeries. The cottage hospital staff did me proud, teasing me with various bits of equipment suitable for geriatric use. My partners gave me a lovely painting of our parish church and the surgery staff also did me proud with a wonderful leaving party which included a treasure chest full of things that amusingly related to a life on the ocean waves, with references to seasickness and lifeboats and sundry other teases. An evening that I thoroughly enjoyed, and will always cherish.

This may hurt a little...

About the Author

Dr Jeremy Bradshaw-Smith was born in Bakewell, Derbyshire in 1934, in the house of his GP grandfather. Before the age of one, he moved to India. His father died in World War II, having been wounded twice in World War I. Dr Jeremy was back in England in 1944, and started at Wellington College in 1947 as a Foundationer (due to his soldier father's death). He studied at St Thomas' Hospital from 1952-1958, gaining his MB BS qualifications, before marrying Ann in 1958. They went on to have four children.

Dr Jeremy did army service from 1959-1963, gained a Diploma in Tropical Disease, and spent one and a half years in East Africa. Back at St Thomas' Hospital, he worked in Obstetrics, gaining a DObst RCOB (Obstetric diploma).

Dr Jeremy started his general practice career in 1964, and was concerned with pioneering computer medical record-keeping.

He retired in 1994, and sailed across the Atlantic with Ann.